The Coconut Oil Handbook: How to Lose Weight, Improve Cholesterol, Alleviate Allergies, Renew Your Skin, and Get Healthier with Coconut Oil

by Jamie Wright

Disclaimer:

The information contained in this book is for general information purposes only. This book is sold with the understanding the author and/or publisher is not giving medical advice, nor should the information contained in this book replace medical advice, nor is it intended to diagnose or treat any disease, illness or other medical condition. Always consult your medical practitioner before making any dietary changes or treating or attempting to treat any medical condition. Reading the information in this book does not create a physician-patient relationship and should not take the place of professional medical advice.

While we endeavor to keep the information up to date and correct, we make no representations or warranties of any kind, express or implied, about the completeness, accuracy, reliability, suitability or availability with respect to the book or the information, products, services, or related graphics contained book for any purpose. Any reliance you place on such information is therefore strictly at your own risk.

Dedication:

This book is dedicated to all those who have made the switch to coconut oil and all those who are thinking about making the switch. I switched over a few years ago and haven't looked back since.

Contents

Coconut Oil: Is It Really All It's Cracked Up to Be?

For many years, coconut oil was written off as being unhealthy by health experts who were quick to point out the high levels of saturated fat it features. Most of these experts will never admit it, but it looks like they were way off base with their wild claims about how bad coconut oil is for the human body.

Study after study has shown the natural saturated fats in coconut oil to be good for the body.

A growing number of people are making use of coconut oil both in the kitchen and as a natural health and beauty product. The fatty acids found in coconut oil are easy to digest and the body processes them quickly, sending them to the liver where they're broken down into smaller units and used for energy.

Once inside the body coconut oil goes to work immediately. It has been shown to lower bad cholesterol, fight off viral infections (including influenza), reduce waist size and kill off bacteria and parasites. Seeing a list of the health benefits of coconut oil may lead one to ask the question, "Is there anything coconut oil doesn't do?" I can answer that for you. Coconut oil doesn't automatically make you skinny and healthy, like some people would have you believe. It's a great start, but it isn't going to get you where you want to be on its own.

Coconut oil is a worthy replacement for a number of other so-called "healthy" vegetable oils. I used parentheses in the previous sentence because many of the vegetable oils people have been led to believe are healthy are anything but. They contain large fat molecules and trans fats that are difficult for the body to process and are more likely to be converted to body fat than the saturated fat found in coconut oil.

In addition to being more than capable in the kitchen, coconut oil also works well for a number of other applications. It works well as a base oil for skin and hair care products and can be applied topically to help ease the effects of a vast array of skin conditions. From athlete's foot to yeast infections, coconut oil has seen use as an effective natural remedy.

This handy oil has so many health benefits some experts have called it a "miracle oil." Those in the know can attest to its many powers, and new uses are constantly being discovered. It's a safe and effective natural remedy for a number of ailment and illnesses, it contributes to good health and it gives your body a quick and effective energy boost.

Coconut oil is all it's cracked up to be and then some. It isn't just a snake oil being sold by merchants looking to cash in on other people's misfortune. It's good stuff, and the science behind it is solid. By the time you finish this book, you're probably going to end up wondering why coconut oil is largely ignored in Western diets. I've often wondered that myself.

There are very few people who couldn't benefit from coconut oil. Read on to find out what tens of thousands of people already know. Coconut oil isn't what you think it is.

It's much better.

The Only Kind of Coconut Oil You Should Use

There's only one kind of coconut oil you should be eating, and that's virgin coconut oil. True virgin coconut oil has the following qualities:

- **It has no additives.**
- **It hasn't been deodorized.**
- **It hasn't been hydrogenated or partially-hydrogenated.**
- **It hasn't undergone any heat treatment.**
- **It isn't bleached.**
- **It isn't made from genetically modified crops.**
- **It's unrefined.**
- **No chemicals have been used in the extraction process.**

Virgin coconut oil is extracted using clean extraction methods like milling, grating or centrifuges. The oil is removed from the coconut in a manner that doesn't use chemicals and nothing is added to or removed from the oil during processing.

While other methods and processes can leave behind trace amounts of nasty chemicals like hexane, virgin coconut oil is created in manner that keeps it pure, hence the use of the word "virgin." You may see the terms "expeller-pressed" and "cold-pressed" used in place of the word "virgin." These oils are not always of the same quality as virgin coconut oil and should generally be avoided.

Unless an oil specifically states on the label that it's virgin, your best bet is to assume it isn't. Virgin coconut oil is highly sought after and is more expensive than other varieties of coconut oil, so there's no way a manufacturer is going to pass up the chance to label their oil as "virgin."

You may come across oils that are labeled as "extra virgin." There are no regulations that lay out the difference between virgin and extra virgin oils. This appears to be a marketing ploy more than anything else. There is rarely anything separating most extra virgin oils from the quality virgin oils on the market.

The key difference between virgin oil and refined oil lies in how each of the types of coconut oil are processed.

Refined coconut oil goes through a number of processing steps that seek to remove taste and smell from the oil. High heat, chemical bleaching and deodorizing and any number of other processes are used to create an oil that's doesn't smell or taste like coconut. The problem with the refining process is it damages the oil and can leave behind trace amounts of the chemicals used during processing. You get oil that is devoid of coconut taste and scent, but is also devoid of many of the benefits of using coconut oil in the first place.

Given the choice between virgin and refined coconut oil, virgin oil is almost always the best choice. That said, if I had to choose between using refined coconut oil and switching to another type of vegetable oil, I'd go with the refined coconut oil.

Partially-hydrogenated coconut oil is the worst kind of coconut on the market because it contains the bad stuff you're trying to get away from by switching to coconut oil. The hydrogenation process creates trans fat where before there was none. We'll discuss trans fat in depth later on in this book, but for now all you need to know is you don't want it in your coconut oil.

If you can afford the extra cost, organic virgin coconut oil is even better.

Organic oil comes from coconut plantations where no chemicals or pesticides are used on the trees the coconuts come from. Trace amounts of pesticides can be passed into coconut oil when the trees are sprayed. Given a choice, I always opt for organic oil. That said, if I had to choose between using nonorganic coconut oil and not using coconut oil at all, I think the health benefits outweigh the risks of nonorganic coconut oil having trace amounts of pesticides in it.

Go with what you can afford and find in your area and you'll be fine.

Our Rapidly Expanding Waistlines: What's Really Going On

We've been hearing for years how bad coconut oil is for us. It's been labeled as being "bad" oil by health agencies that scream and yell and jump up and down as they point the finger at saturated fat. They're quick to point to early studies done in the 1960's that at first glance seem to prove coconut oil raises cholesterol levels.

The problem with the studies being referenced is the experts largely fail to point out one glaring flaw. The oil used in the lion's share of these early studies was hydrogenated coconut oil. Hydrogenated oil of any kind is bad, so it stands to reason that hydrogenated coconut oil would be bad as well.

Before we get into hydrogenation and why it's bad, let's back up a bit and take a look at a group of people who consume coconut oil regularly and have for thousands of years. Pacific Islanders consume coconuts and coconut oil as a key part of their diet. It's a dietary staple and makes up a large percentage of the fat they consume. If what we've been taught about the saturated fats in coconut oil is true, this should be an unhealthy group of people as a whole. Clogged arteries and heart attacks should abound. Their cholesterol should be off the charts and they should be overweight, sick and dropping like flies.

The reality is far from what you'd expect. These people are healthier than we are as a nation. They have good cardiovascular health and do not have elevated blood cholesterol levels. They live long healthy lives free of many of the health problems plaguing the Western world.

Don't get me wrong. Coconut oil isn't the only reason these populations are healthy. They generally eat clean diets with minimal amounts of fried and processed food and they're highly active. Even so, if coconut oil is as bad as some would have you believe, there'd be more heart disease than there is, even with their healthier lifestyle factored in.

There's no doubt that there's a real obesity problem in America right now. If you're living in America, that probably comes as no surprise. All you have to do is look around you when you're out and about to see how bad things are. Overweight people abound, and there are a growing number of obese and morbidly obese people tipping the scales at weights approaching that of a small car.

The next time you're at the mall or, better yet, at a fast food chain, take a look around you. How many people do you see that look healthy? A few? None at all? Now count the people who are carrying a few extra pounds and then the people who are obese. It's estimated that more than 70% of Americans are overweight and more than 60% are classified as obese. I think that estimate may be too low.

The fact that you're reading this book is a good start.

It shows you're being proactive about learning how to lose weight and stay healthy. That's a lot more than most Americans care to do—and food manufacturers and grocery stores know this. Instead of selling healthy foods that are designed to work *with* the human body to promote good health, most grocery stores sell unhealthy foods that are made with products that bear little resemblance to the foods our grandparents ate when they were kids.

In fact, many of the foods consumed in the Western world are so processed that manufacturers have to add scent and flavor back into them to make them recognizable. If you saw what the food you're eating looks like before it's returned to a semi-normal state, you'd be sick to your stomach. You're putting poison in your body that's masquerading as real food.

Not convinced? Read the label on that pack of cookies or that processed cheese you're eating. I'll bet you don't have a clue what half of the stuff in your food is there for. You're consuming a cocktail of chemicals added to your food to make it last longer and to get it to the store as cheaply and as quickly as possible. It doesn't benefit you to have synthetic additives, dyes and nitrates added to your food. It benefits the bottom line of the manufacturers.

And to be honest with you, it's our own fault. Most of us don't give a damn about our health, so why should food manufacturers? We've allowed them to poison us for years, happily eating garbage more fit for the trash heap than it is the dinner table. Things weren't always this way. Less than half a century ago, waistlines were much smaller. The obesity rate was hovering right around 10% and the amount of people who were overweight was much lower. The average American was in shape and much healthier, as a result.

So what happened?

I'll tell you what. Hydrogenated oils happened.

That's right—the rise in popularity of hydrogenated oils and processed foods largely tracks the ever-increasing size of the average American's pants. We stopped caring what was put in our food in the name of convenience and are to this day willingly sacrificing our health for a quick and easy—and let's not forget, inexpensive—meal. Instead of reading ingredient lists, we check the microwave instructions to see how easy the garbage we're buying will be to prepare. Instead of checking to see if our lunchtime snack contains poisons and carcinogens, we think we're going above and beyond if we check to see how many calories it has in it.

If one were to hop in a time machine and take a TV dinner and a variety of other processed foods back a couple hundred years in time to try to serve it to our forefathers, we'd be laughed out of the dining room. A fast food cheeseburger today barely resembles the burgers of old. What passes for food now would have been met with derision from our not-so-distant ancestors.

Hydrogenated oils are largely to blame for this change. In order to understand why, let's take a look at what hydrogenated oils are and why they're so heavily used today.

The hydrogenation process involves passing hydrogen bubbles through heated oil in order to get the hydrogen to bond with the fatty acids in the oil. This process is usually stopped before all of fatty acids bond with hydrogen molecules, leaving behind partially-hydrogenated oil that's the consistency of butter, but costs a fraction of what butter costs to produce or buy. Manufacturers get the flavor and texture of butter at a much lower price point, plus they get the added bonus of a longer shelf life.

It's a win-win situation for those making and selling the food. They get food that tastes the same—and in some cases, better—than food produced with real butter. The food lasts longer, so they can produce more of it and leave it sitting on store shelves for a longer period of time before it goes rancid. This all equals more money lining the pockets of manufacturers and the grocery stores that buy from them.

The problem with this new substance created through hydrogenation is that while it has a similar taste and texture to butter or other animal fats, the similarities end there. The hydrogenation process creates trans fats, which are the most dangerous kind of fat to put in your body. Those who consume it often end up paying a steep price. Trans fats raise the level of bad cholesterol in your body and clog your arteries, amongst a number of other health problems they've been shown to cause.

Trans fat has been clinically proven to pack on the pounds. One study showed trans fat not only makes you gain weight, it also moves the fat you're already carrying to your abdominal area (1).

Eliminating trans fats from your diet will go a long way toward ensuring longevity and is a great start down the road to getting eating better and getting fit. The problem with cutting out trans fats is it's easier said than done.

Around 40% of the food sold in stores today contains trans fats. The following types of food are the biggest offenders:

- **Cakes.**
- **Chips.**
- **Cookies.**
- **Fast food.**
- **Frosting.**
- **Frozen pizza.**
- **Junk food.**
- **Margarines and butter imitations.**
- **Packaged baked goods.**
- **Pies.**
- **Processed foods.**
- **Vegetable shortening.**

The list goes on and on. Walk the middle aisles of a grocery store and you'll see row after row of unhealthy foods.

Trans fats are everywhere and most people don't bother to even look at the label of the foods they're eating to see if they're in there. Those who do glance at the label may be lulled into a false sense of security. Food companies are allowed to list zero grams of trans fat on the label of their foods as long as they have less than half a gram of trans fat per serving.

Let that sink in for a moment. Reread it if you'd like.

Manufacturers can legally label foods as being free of trans fat even when there's trans fat in them.

A half gram of trans fat doesn't sound like a lot until you look at what passes for a serving of most foods. Serving sizes are much smaller than you'd expect. A single serving of breakfast cereal barely covers the bottom of the bowl. A single serving of chips is a small handful. It isn't uncommon for people to eat 2 to 3 servings in a single sitting and think nothing of it. If you eat 2 servings of a food that contains just under 0.5g of trans fat, you've just eaten nearly a gram of trans fat without realizing it. If you do that with 3 or 4 different foods a day that you think are free of trans fat, you could be slowly killing yourself without even realizing what you're doing.

So what can be done?

For one, you need to start reading the labels on the packaged foods you buy. Don't just look to see whether the food items you're buying have trans fat in them. You now know that you're being lied to. Instead, you need to check the ingredients to see whether there are ingredients in the food that you know to have trans fats.

Here are some of the biggest offenders when it comes to trans fat:

- **Any ingredient that has the words "hydrogenated" or "partially-hydrogenated."** Fully hydrogenated oils don't contain high levels of trans fat because most of the fat has been hydrogenated. The reason I included hydrogenated ingredients on the list is because there's a chance a manufacturer will list an ingredient as hydrogenated when it's only partially hydrogenated. Some manufacturers use the two terms interchangeably.

- **Canola oil.**
- **Diglycerides.**
- **Margarine.**
- **Modified oil.**
- **Monodiglycerides.**
- **Shortening.**
- **Triglycerides.**
- **Vegetable fat.**
- **Vegetable shortening.**

Keep in mind that you're going to have to be extremely careful about watching what you eat to eliminate trans fats from your diet. Restaurants, delis, bakeries and fast food joints all may have food on the menu that contains trans fats. Don't be afraid to ask what type of oil is used in the food you're buying. If partially hydrogenated oil is used, it has trans fats in it.

You're also going to have to monitor what type of oil is used to cook your foods.

Vegetable oils that don't normally contain trans fat have been shown to form trans fat at high temperatures like those used to fry foods. The amount of trans fat formed in a single use isn't high, but oil that's reused many times over can contain large amounts of trans fats. The more the oil is used, the more trans fat it will contain. At home you should change your cooking oil frequently. When eating out it doesn't hurt to ask how often the oil is changed—but don't expect an honest answer. Most restaurant owners aren't going to tell you they've been using the same oil for a month.

The only honest way to make sure you aren't getting unnecessary trans fat and hydrogenated oils is to make your food at home from raw ingredients. Switch from partially-hydrogenated oils in your foods and baked goods to an oil like coconut oil that doesn't contain dangerous trans fat.

It's best to avoid fried foods altogether, but we all know that probably isn't going to happen. Instead of using partially-hydrogenated oils or vegetable oils with low smoke points that may cause trans fats to form under high heat, make the switch to coconut oil, which has a high enough smoke point that trans fats aren't a concern unless you repeatedly reuse the same oil.

Whatever you do, don't switch from another oil over to partially-hydrogenated coconut oil. That's like kicking a crack habit so you can start shooting heroin. You're exchanging one bad oil for another. Stick to pure unrefined coconut oil and your body will be much better off.

What You Need to Know About Cholesterol

Before we get too far into this book, we need to have a little discussion about cholesterol. What I'm about to tell you may come as a surprise unless you've dug deep to get the real scoop on cholesterol.

Cholesterol is produced naturally by your body and is needed for a number of bodily functions. Your body uses cholesterol for the following important tasks, amongst other things:

- **Bile production.**
- **Cell health and strength.**
- **Digestion.**
- **Healthy skin.**
- **Keeps bones flexible.**
- **Nerve function.**
- **Promotes healthy brain function.**
- **To produce hormones.**
- **Vitamin D production.**

Cholesterol isn't all bad. Your body needs cholesterol and your liver produces it on a mass scale.

The food you eat doesn't impact the cholesterol level in your body nowhere near as much as you probably think it does. Dietary cholesterol accounts for maybe 10% of your blood cholesterol levels. It would take a lot of cholesterol-rich food to have a significant impact on your overall cholesterol level.

If you fail to eat foods with cholesterol in them, your cholesterol levels can actually begin to increase. Your body will try to adjust its cholesterol levels to account for the lack of dietary cholesterol you're taking in and it may overshoot. Eating foods with natural cholesterol like eggs and meats can help lower your blood cholesterol levels.

When it comes to foods that increase cholesterol, saturated fat is fairly low on the totem pole. This may come as a surprise, as we've been told for years that saturated fat causes dangerous spikes in cholesterol.

Carbohydrates and sugars are the real problem, as they can increase LDL cholesterol while decreasing HDL cholesterol. The insulin the body produces to deal with rise in blood sugar associated with eating simple carbohydrates can cause your cholesterol to go up. Foods that are high in carbohydrates and hydrogenated fats and oils are the real culprits when it comes to cholesterol, not natural saturated fat.

HDL cholesterol is touted as good cholesterol and LDL is labeled as bad. Most people's understanding of cholesterol ends there.

LDL cholesterol carries cholesterol through your blood and transports it across your body. They're considered the "bad boy" of the cholesterol world because they can oxidize and form plaque in your arteries. HDL cholesterol molecules are smaller cholesterol molecules that bring unused cholesterol to your liver. They help prevent the formation of plaque in your arteries and are found in higher levels in healthy people.

There's evidence that seems to indicate high cholesterol may not be as deadly as we've been lead to believe.

A University of Connecticut study done in 2012 looked at dietary cholesterol and its impact on coronary heart disease in countries where there is no top-end recommended limit on cholesterol intake and concluded that the evidence "supports the notion that the recommendations limiting dietary cholesterol should be reconsidered" (2). That's a strong statement that stands in stark contrast to conventional knowledge of cholesterol.

A Yale study done in 1994 looked at 997 elderly adults and attempted to associate high serum cholesterol with coronary heart disease mortality. The study wasn't able to make the association and further failed to link high serum cholesterol levels to overall mortality rates (3). Think about this for a moment. As far as studies go, a group approaching 1,000 people is a large group. The fact that the entire group was elderly should have meant that high serum cholesterol levels would affect them more than it would a healthy young adult. Instead, this study showed no correlation between serum cholesterol levels and death rates.

Perhaps even more telling is the fact that despite cholesterol-lowering drugs being prescribed at an unprecedented rate, more than a million people in the United States alone will have heart attacks this year and around 600,000 people will die from heart disease. And this is in a nation that heavily prescribes drugs to control cholesterol—to the tune of $30 billion or so dollars' worth of prescription medications a year. There's big bucks being spent on cholesterol management, but the money doesn't seem to be buying a life spend free of heart trouble.

A study done in Finland looked at 3,490 men to test the effectiveness of cardiovascular disease prevention. The trial lasted for 5 years and the results were surprising. Heart disease risk was lowered in the group that underwent preventative treatment, which is what you'd expect. What wasn't expected was the increase in both total deaths and cardiac deaths. There were 34 cardiac deaths in the intervention group and only 14 in the control group (4).

This begs the question why we've been lead down the wrong path for so many years. The answer is more complicated than simply saying "money" and leaving it at that. There are very few health experts who would intentionally mislead people when it comes to something that could potentially cost them their life. Doctors are taught from an early age about the evils of cholesterol and are told statin drugs are safe and will lower cholesterol, so they prescribe them at the first sign of high cholesterol.

Companies come up with products that "may" or "should" lower your risk of heart disease. Their products work for some people, while leaving others out in the cold. Some of these foods and products work well. A number of them don't, or they do, but carry potentially dangerous side effects. While there are some people who need drugs to regulate their cholesterol, there are quite a few with prescriptions they don't really need.

In many cases, it's probably best to let the body work naturally, producing the cholesterol it needs as it goes. Instead of prescribing expensive medications, a more holistic approach may be a much better option. Cholesterol can often be regulated naturally; it just takes more work to watch what you eat and to live a healthier lifestyle.

How to Use Coconut Oil to Improve Cholesterol

Let's clear up a common misconception right away. The saturated fats in virgin coconut oil do not negatively impact your cholesterol. Those firmly in the "all saturated fats are bad camp" refuse to look at the facts and discount any study that proves this to be correct. The scientific evidence appears to show that all saturated fats are not created equally and the saturated fat in coconut oil stands head and shoulders above the rest.

Consuming virgin coconut oil can raise the total amount of serum cholesterol in your blood. This isn't necessarily a bad thing, and it surely isn't a good measure of whether your cholesterol is at a healthy level or not. A better measure is the ratio of bad LDL cholesterol to good HDL cholesterol. This is indicative of whether your body has the proper cholesterol balance and is functioning at a healthy level. A total serum cholesterol increase isn't a bad thing when it's the HDL cholesterol that's increasing. When you look at the ratio of bad to good cholesterol, coconut oil has a positive impact because it increases good cholesterol and therefore improves the cholesterol ratio in the blood. A total increase in cholesterol as a whole isn't bad when your ratio of bad to good cholesterol improves as a result.

If saturated fat intake from coconut oil is as bad as some health agencies would have you believe, it would stand to reason that populations that consume large amounts of coconut oil would have higher cholesterol levels and, as a result, would see an increase in heart disease. Studies of populations across the globe that consume high levels of coconut oil as a staple in their diet have been shown to be healthier, on average, than those consuming Western diets with limited saturated fat. Total cholesterol levels do indeed increase with consumption of coconut oil, but that increase is tied to HDL cholesterol gains, which improves the LDL:HDL ratio.

In a study of 1,839 Filipino women, researchers found that coconut oil intake increased HDL cholesterol levels and "was not significantly associated with" an increase in LDL cholesterol levels (5). Another study of the Minangkabau population of West Sumatra determined that consumption of saturated fat, including large amounts of coconut oil, was not a predictor of coronary heart disease (6).

In yet another study, one group of women was given 30mL of soybean oil a day, while another group was given 30mL of coconut oil, and at the end of a 12-week period, the group that was given the coconut oil had higher levels of HDL cholesterol in the blood and their LDL:HDL ratio improved. The soybean oil group showed decreased HDL cholesterol levels in the blood, an increase in total cholesterol and an increase in the LDL:HDL ratio. The coconut oil group also saw a reduction in waist circumference that wasn't realized by the soybean oil group (7).

Lowering bad serum cholesterol may be as simple as making the switch from other vegetable oils to coconut oil. While coconut oil does indeed raise overall serum cholesterol levels in most people, it raises the good HDL cholesterol more than it raises LDL cholesterol. This improves the blood cholesterol ratio, which is the true determinant of cholesterol health in the body.

That is, if you believe cholesterol is to blame for heart problems at all. A growing number of experts are going on record stating cholesterol may not be the enemy of the heart we've been lead to believe it is.

The Many Faces of Fat

Let's take a moment to discuss fats and the role they play in the human body. The information in this chapter is key to understanding the rest of the book, so pay close attention.

Fats and oils are scientifically referred to as lipids. If a lipid solidifies at room temperature, it is classified as a fat. If it is liquid, it is considered an oil. All fats are not the same, and a single fat can be made up of a number of chemical compounds. The chemical composition differs from fat to fat and can even differ between fats of the same type. For example, pastured animals that are allowed to roam free and graze on grass will have different compounds in their fat than will animals that are raised in pens and fed the same thing day in and day out.

Let's get one thing clear. Regardless of what you've been told, fat in and of itself isn't a bad thing in your diet.

Fat is an essential part of your diet and is required by your body to do things like process certain vitamins and control insulin levels. Lipids are required by the body to process vitamins A, D, E and K, which are called fat-soluble vitamins. Lipids also play an important role in making you feel full, which is important because that's your body's way of knowing when to stop eating.

The main role fats play in the human body is to provide an alternate source of energy so the body doesn't start burning the proteins it needs to build and repair tissue cells. When there's a shortage of fats and carbohydrates, proteins are consumed for energy and there aren't as many available for the body to use to rebuild tissue.

There are 3 basic types of fat:

- **Saturated fats.**
- **Unsaturated fat.**
- **Trans fat.**

Let's take a closer look at each type.

Saturated Fats

Saturated fats are fat molecules that have hydrogen molecules attached at every location one can be attached at. They're "saturated" with hydrogen molecules. For now, that's all you need to know about saturated fats. We'll cover them more in the next chapter.

Unsaturated Fats

In unsaturated fats, some of the hydrogen molecules are absent. The fat molecules aren't completely saturated with hydrogen.

There are two basic types of unsaturated fats:

- **Monounsaturated fats.** These fats are missing a pair of hydrogen atoms.
- **Polyunsaturated fats.** These fats have two or more pairs of hydrogen missing.

Monounsaturated fats have low melting points and are liquid at room temperature, but are usually solid when cooled down. They're widely touted by health experts as being healthy fats and are found in high amounts in seeds, nuts and in vegetable oils like canola, olive, avocado and peanut oil. They're also found in meats and dairy products.

Polyunsaturated fats are unsaturated fats that are liquid no matter what the temperature. They're commonly found in corn, soybean and sunflower oil, as well as certain nuts and seeds and cold-water fish. They're also touted by health experts as being good fats.

The problem with polyunsaturated fatty acids (PUFAs) (and monounsaturated fats, to a lesser extent) is they tend to be less stable than saturated fats. The more hydrogen atoms they're missing, the less stable they are. Unsaturated fats are more susceptible to oxidation and free radical damage, which can lead to all sorts of problems at the cellular level. Cancer, inflammation, wrinkles, hormonal imbalance, you name it. All are thought to be tied to free radical damage.

That's right, folks. The same oils you've been led to believe are healthy may be anything but.

Scientific studies are beginning to show evidence that unsaturated fats aren't all they're cracked up to be. Here are just a few of the studies that seem to prove saturated fat may not be the knight in shining armor health experts have made it out to be:

- In a 1994 study published in the Lancet Medical Journal, researchers from the Wynn Institute for Metabolic Research found dietary polyunsaturated fats make up 74% of the plaque found in clogged arteries (8).
- A 2012 report published by the Department of Internal Medicine at Charles University in the Czech Republic implicated polyunsaturated fat as playing a role in triggering some psychiatric diseases (9).
- In an analysis of prostate cancer cases registered with the European Prospective Investigation into Cancer and Nutrition (EPIC), the Center for Cardiovascular Research at Aarhus University

Hospital in Denmark concluded that PUFAs may be related to prostate cancer (10).

After reading this, you may be tempted to completely eliminate unsaturated fats from your diet. That isn't necessary and would be nearly impossible because most foods contain at least some amount of unsaturated fat in them. Small amounts of unsaturated fat aren't bad for you because your body needs the omega-6 fatty acids they're made up of.

The problem with most Western diets is consumption of unsaturated fats is taken to the extreme. A number of experts recommend keeping the omega-3 fatty acid to omega-6 fatty acid ratio at somewhere near 1:1 because that's the ratio the human body evolved on. That means for every unit of omega-6 fatty acids you're getting from unsaturated fat, you should be getting 1 unit of omega-3 fatty acids from saturated fat.

Historically, a 1:1 ratio has been the norm. It wasn't until the last hundred years or so that things really started to change.

According to information published in a study by the Center for Genetics, Nutrition and Health in Washington D.C., the ratio of omega-3 to omega-6 in Western diets is 1:15 to 1:16.7 (11). That's a huge difference, and it could be impacting your health. Lowering your ratio of omega-3 to omega-6 fatty acids decreases your susceptibility to cardiovascular disease, cancer and a number of other diseases you don't want ravaging your body.

I'll finish this section with a thought that's based more on anecdotal evidence than actual science.

I live in the country and there are more than a few pig farms in my area. In fact, I have good friends who raise pigs. I was more than a little surprised to find out that pig farmers supplement their pigs' diets with vegetable oils that are packed with unsaturated fats like canola, corn and soybean oil to fatten them up. When I asked whether they'd tried feeding the pigs coconut oil, the farmer looked at me like I was crazy and said it wouldn't work.

Coconut oil was experimented with in the 1940s as a possible livestock fattener by farmers looking to cut costs by making the switch from expensive and dangerous drugs to an inexpensive oil. Coconut oil didn't fatten the cows they fed it to. Instead, it left them lean and made them more active. Fast forward 75 years and farmers still know what most people don't. Vegetable oils high in unsaturated fats pack on the pounds while coconut oil doesn't.

Trans Fats

While there's much debate regarding saturated and unsaturated fats and which is better for the human body, there's one type of fat everyone can agree is bad—and that's trans fat. We touched upon trans fat in the last chapter, but let's take another look at this deadly fat.

Trans fat is formed during the hydrogenation process, which is a man-made process through which unsaturated oils are saturated with hydrogen. This process allows manufacturers to create oils that act like saturated fats from inexpensive vegetable oils. Trans fat is formed when the hydrogenation process is stopped midstream to create partially-hydrogenated oil, which contain a mixture of fats that are solid at room temperature, but melt when warmed up. Partially-hydrogenated oils are created and used by manufacturers because they most closely resemble animal fats like butter and are less prone to going rancid. When a manufacturer can save money and is able to keep food products on the shelves longer, who cares what it's doing to the people who eat it?

Well, for one, you should care.

Your body doesn't recognize trans fat once it enters the body and is unable to metabolize them. While the exact reasons why trans fat is so damaging aren't completely understood, all experts agree they're bad for you. Really bad.

If you only take one thing from this book, understand that trans fat is in your food to extend shelf-life and nothing else. It isn't going to extend your life . . . and may end up cutting it drastically short.

Man-made trans fat is damaged fat that does damage on a large scale once it enters the body. Each teaspoon of trans fat-laden oil that you consume does a little bit of damage, and eventually the damage adds up to a crisis event like an artery blockage that leads to a heart attack or stroke. Consuming hydrogenated fats is like putting regular gas in a car with a diesel engine. The car may run for a while, but it isn't running on the fuel it's designed to run on and will quickly start to wear down.

Trans fat has been linked to the following health risks:

- **Cancer.** While there haven't been any definitive studies linking trans fat to cancer, there is evidence that indicates it may raise the risk of certain types of cancer like breast and prostate cancer.
- **Coronary heart disease.** It's estimated that between 30,000 and 100,000 cardiac deaths per year in the United States alone are due to trans fat consumption.
- **Diabetes.** Studies tying diabetes to consumption of trans fat are conflicting, but there is evidence that appears to link trans fats to type 2 diabetes, which is the most common type of diabetes (12).
- **It increases the level of bad cholesterol in the blood while lowering good cholesterol.** Remember that bad to good cholesterol level? Trans fat impacts it negatively.
- **Mental health issues.** Trans fats increase your risk of developing serious depressive disorders and may be tied to the onset of Alzheimer's Disease.
- **Weight gain.** Consumption of trans fat has been shown to increase waist size and abdominal fat (1). Trans fat is stored by the body as body fat at a faster pace than other types of fat.

Trans fat is so bad it's been banned in a number of nations. Denmark, Iceland and Austria have all effectively banned trans fats from foods. In the United States, there are some cities and counties where trans fat isn't allowed in fast food, but the only national laws on the books regulate how packaged foods with trans fats have to be labeled. The amount of trans fat a food contains has to be on the label, with one big concession to manufacturers.

Surprisingly, foods with less than 0.5 grams of trans fat per serving can be labeled as having 0 trans fat. What this means is you could be eating trans fats in your diet as we speak, without ever knowing it if you trust that the nutritional information is correct. If you consume a lot of processed or restaurant foods, you could easily be exceeding the 2 gram per day top end limit on trans fat consumption recommended by the American Heart Association, and you'd never know it.

While eliminating unsaturated fats from your diet isn't possible—and isn't desirable since your body does need some unsaturated fat to survive—you should eliminate as much trans fat from your diet as you can.

More and more people are realizing the ill effects trans fats have on the human body. Sadly, a lot of these people are realizing it when they're struck with any number of illnesses related to overconsumption of trans fat.

In an attempt to get around the stigma (and labeling requirement) associated with trans fat, manufacturers are using a relatively new type of fat called interesterified fat. The interesterification process creates a new type of fat that, like trans fat, isn't recognized by the human body. While the verdict is still out on interesterified fats, there is evidence indicating they aren't good for you either. A 2007 study showed interesterified fats to have a similar effect on cholesterol and blood glucose as trans fat (13).

To avoid interesterified fats, you're going to have to look at the ingredient list. Anything with the words "stearic," stearate," or "interesterified" should be avoided. Better yet, just eat natural or raw foods that haven't been processed or altered in any way. You'll largely avoid trans fats *and* interesterified fats and you'll be all the more healthy for it.

The Coconut Oil Saturated Fat Myth

When most people first hear about coconut oil and its many health benefits, the first thing they do is turn to their favorite search engine and do a search for "coconut oil." The results can be a little disconcerting to say the least. There's about a 50-50 split between sites claiming coconut oil is the best thing since sliced bread (cooked with coconut oil, of course) and sites claiming it's the devil in disguise because of the saturated fat it contains.

This begs the question why is there such a great divide between differing groups of people who appear to be working toward the same goal.

The Western world's disdain for saturated fats largely comes from a study by Ancel Keys in the 50's where he appeared to tie death rates in multiple countries to consumption of saturated fat (14). He compared nations like the United States, where high levels of saturated fats are consumed, with nations like Japan, where saturated fat consumption is very low and made the connection between heart disease mortality and saturated fats. All of the nations included in his study seemed to support the theory that saturated fats are a leading cause of heart disease.

There's a major problem with this study, and it's one that's rarely pointed out. It appears that Keys cherry-picked the nations he used in his study. There were a number of other nations for which the information Keys used was available, and for those nations the picture becomes less clear. The study also failed to factor in other variables, like the fact that the Japanese are more active as a nation and tend to consume healthier foods that are lower in sugar.

Combine Keys' data with lobbying from the edible oils industry and all of a sudden saturated fats are left out in the cold. Health agencies jumped on the bandwagon and saturated fat was demonized.

Fast forward to 2006 and the Women's Health Initiative study appears to leave the theory that saturated fats are tied to heart disease dead in the water. In the largest low-fat diet study ever recorded, more than 48,000 women were monitored for an average of just over 8 years. The study found that eating a diet low in total fat (and in saturated fat, as a result) had no effect on heart disease (15). That's right, there was nothing linking saturated fat with heart disease.

So what then of the oft-cited studies that seem to show coconut oil is bad for your cholesterol? It appears that at least some of these studies are more than a bit misleading in that they used partially-hydrogenated coconut oil instead of virgin coconut oil. The studies that use virgin coconut oil typically show it to be cholesterol neutral or to reduce the ratio of bad to good cholesterol, which is beneficial to the body.

In his 1992 Framingham Heart Study, William P. Castelli, M.D., found that the more saturated fat, cholesterol and calories people take in, the lower their serum cholesterol is (16). Other studies have found people who switch from coconut oil to other oils see their cholesterol levels rise and people who start using coconut oil see their cholesterol drop. This stands in stark contrast to what we've taught about saturated fat.

Coconut oil is nearly 90% saturated fat, but it's largely made up of medium-chain fatty acids (MCFAs). These fatty acids aren't circulated through the blood in the same manner the long-chain fatty acids (LCFAs) are, so there's little chance of them being stored as body fat. LCFAs require special processing and are harder for the body to break down. They're sent out into the bloodstream and travel through the body, where they're more likely to be stored as fat.

MCFAs only enter the bloodstream for a short period of time. They're broken down and sent directly to the liver through a vein known as the portal vein, which connects the intestines to the liver. MCFAs are easily digested and are much more likely to be used as energy than they are to be turned into body fat.

While you probably won't live to see most health experts do an about-face on coconut oil or saturated fats, there are a lot of studies that indicate saturated fats—and the saturated fats in coconut oil in particular—got a bad rap. Coconut oil can be part of a healthy diet. It is for millions of people the world over, many of which are healthier because of it.

So, What about "Healthy" Vegetable Oils & Margarines?

Vegetable oils and margarines are often touted as "heart-healthy" alternatives to butter and oils that contain saturated fats. The problem is the science behind these oils largely fails to prove these claims to be true.

These so-called "healthy" oils are derived by heavily processing the seeds of the plants they come from. Many of the oils are chemically extracted and the most-used oils are partially-hydrogenated, which makes them even more toxic to the body. The seeds the oils are extracted from often come from genetically-modified hybrid seeds that have been treated with pesticides and chemical fertilizers.

It isn't just the plants that the oils are derived from that are bathed in chemicals.

Petroleum solvents are often used in the extraction process and chemicals and acids are used to treat, deodorize and change the color of the oil. Hydrogenation or partial-hydrogenation does even more damage, because this is the step in which trans fats are added to the oil. The vegetable oil or butter replacement you get as a final product is so far removed from the original pure oil that it's practically unrecognizable.

The human body isn't designed to properly process most vegetable oils and the chemicals that are added to them. They haven't been around for long enough for the body to adapt to the point where it's able to effectively process large amounts of polyunsaturated fat, let alone any trace amounts of other chemicals the oils contain. Up until the early 1900's the human diet consisted largely of animal fats. We ate meat, butter and lard, and we drank whole milk—and we were healthier on average then than we are now. Our diets then were heavy on omega-3 fatty acids and light on foods containing omega-6 fatty acids.

Now, the ratio of omega-3 to omega-6 in our diets is heavily skewed toward the omega-6 fatty acids found in vegetable oils. We've added large amounts of vegetable oil to our diets, where before they were practically non-existent. According to the USDA, we consumed 9.8 pounds of salad and cooking oils in the 1950's compared to 35.2 pounds in the year 2000. That's roughly a three-fold increase in the amount of cooking oils we're consuming. Total added fat and oil consumption increased nearly 70 percent from the 1950's to the year 2000.

No wonder we're unhealthy as a nation.

The majority of Americans eat whatever they want without paying attention to what's in it—and manufacturers know this. Those of us that do pay attention are being lead to believe vegetable oils are the answer to our cholesterol (and other health) problems, regardless of what a number of studies seem to indicate—and what the decline in our health as a nation tells us.

Butter consumption in 1900 approached 20 pounds per year. Heart disease was 4th on the list of leading causes of death and cancer ranked 8th. Fast forward more than a hundred years and butter and margarine have largely been replaced by "healthy" oils and butter replacements and heart disease is the leading causes of death and cancer sits firmly at number 2 on the list. While the switch to vegetable oils isn't the only cause of this drastic change, it's tough not to believe they're at least partially responsible once you learn about the dangers of these oils.

Oxidation is a big problem when it comes to the polyunsaturated fats found in most vegetable oils. Exposure of these oils to heat, light or oxygen ramps up the rate at which oxidation can occur. Oxidation can also take place in the body.

When oxidation takes place, dangerous free radicals are formed. While there's much debate as to the safety of vegetable oils high in polyunsaturated fats, most experts agree free radicals in the body are never a good thing. They contribute to inflammation and cell damage and are widely believed to promote a number of diseases and ailments, not the least of which are cancer and diabetes.

In a Scottish study published in the European Journal of Clinical Nutrition, researchers found that lipid peroxidation and oxidative stress increased when dietary intake of polyunsaturated fatty acids increased (17).

Because of their propensity for oxidation, manufacturers sometimes add synthetic antioxidant chemicals like butylated hydroxyanisole (BHA) and butylated hydroxytoluene (BHT), which are chemical additives designed to prolong the life of the oil. BHA is thought to be a possible carcinogen and BHT may also be tied to cancer. While there are conflicting studies regarding BHA and BHT and their effect on the body, it's tough to recommend a preservative that's possibly tied to cancer. In addition to being possibly tied to cancer, BHA and BHT have been linked to allergic reactions, dermatitis, headaches, and joint pain and stomach issues in some people.

While the body needs some polyunsaturated fat, it doesn't need it at the levels found in most Western diets. Almost all natural food contains polyunsaturated fat in small amounts. This is all you really need to keep the body functioning the way nature intended. Adding large amounts of oils containing extra polyunsaturated fat overloads the body and ups the chances of oxidative damage.

For those wanting to limit polyunsaturated fat intake, the following oils and fats should be avoided or only consumed in small amounts:

- **Butter substitutes (amount of polyunsaturated fat varies, but tends to be high).**
- **Canola oil (28% polyunsaturated fat).**
- **Corn oil (62% polyunsaturated fat).**
- **Cottonseed oil (52% polyunsaturated fat).**
- **Flaxseed oil (70% to 90% polyunsaturated fat).**
- **Grapeseed oil (70% polyunsaturated fat).**
- **High-linoleic safflower oil (75% polyunsaturated fat).**
- **High-linoleic sunflower oil (40% saturated fat).**
- **Margarine (level of polyunsaturated fat varies).**
- **Peanut oil (32% polyunsaturated fat).**
- **Sesame seed oil (43% polyunsaturated fat).**

- **Soybean oil (58% polyunsaturated fat).**

Coconut oil has large amounts on saturated fat and a small amount of polyunsaturated fat, which makes it a good choice to minimize the effect of free radical damage in the body. This is especially true if you're using cooking oil to fry foods, as unsaturated fats are more prone to oxidative damage during the frying process than saturated fats.

Lauric Acid in Coconut Oil

We've already touched upon medium-chain fatty acids (MCFAs) and why they're better for the body than the long-chain fatty acids (LCFAs) found in many vegetable oils. Lauric acid is an MCFA found in abundance in coconut oil. It makes up approximately 50% of the total composition of pure virgin coconut oil.

Virgin coconut oil is one of the most abundant sources of lauric acid found in nature. The only other natural source where it's found in large amounts is in breast milk. It's largely responsible for the difference in health between breast-fed babies and those that are fed formula that doesn't contain lauric acid.

Once lauric acid enters the body it is converted to monolaurin, which has strong antibacterial, antifungal, antiviral and antimicrobial properties. It breaks through the cell walls of bacteria, fungus and viruses, rendering them inert in the process.

Monolaurin has been shown to be an effective treatment for the following bacterial and fungal infections:

- **Athlete's foot.**
- **Candida albicans (yeast infection).**
- **Colds.**
- **Cytomegalovirus (HHV-5).**
- **Flu.**
- **Giardia lamblia.**
- **Hepatitis C.**

- **Herpes.**
- **Listeria monocytogenes.**
- **Measles.**
- **Pneumonovirus.**
- **Ringworm.**
- **Rubeola.**
- **Sarcoma.**
- **Staphylococcus aureus (staph infection).**
- **Streptococcus.**

While antibiotics are the normal prescribed treatment for many of the bacterial infections in the above list, monolaurin is able to inactivate the bacteria without negatively impacting probiotic bacteria in the digestive system. Antibiotics aren't able to effectively target just the bad bacteria in the same manner as monolaurin. They kill all bacteria, including good bacteria, which gives the bad bacteria a chance to regain a foothold one you stop taking the antibiotic. This can lead to superbacteria that are resistant to antibiotics.

There's some evidence that indicates monolaurin inactivates the HIV virus, at least to a certain extent. IN one study, after a 6 month period 7 of 14 patients receiving various levels of monolaurin showed reduced viral loads. 3 of the 7 showed significant reductions (18). While the test group was small, the results are promising and more testing should be in order.

The average Western diet is largely lacking lauric acid. Aside from finding a nursing mother willing to kick you down some breast milk, your only real option for adding natural lauric acid to your diet (and therefore giving your body the ability to produce monolaurin) is through consumption of coconut oil or other products containing coconut. While it isn't known exactly how much monolaurin will be synthesized from the coconut oil, even a small amount can be beneficial.

You get approximately 7 grams of lauric acid per tablespoon of virgin coconut oil. It's recommended by coconut oil experts that most people consume 2 to 3 tablespoons per day. They can be taken as a daily supplement or they can be added to your food.

Reduce Inflammation and Improve Your Health

When taken at face value, the word inflammation doesn't sound all that bad. It's your body's natural response when it senses something isn't right. After all, what's a little inflammation when you've got much worse health issues to worry about?

Well, I've got news for you.

Inflammation doesn't sound like a big deal, but chronic inflammation can cause serious health issues. It has been tied to the following conditions (and more):

- **Acne.**
- **Allergies.**
- **Alzheimer's disease.**
- **Arthritis.**
- **Asthma.**
- **Atherosclerosis.**
- **Autoimmune diseases.**
- **Cancer.**
- **Celiac disease.**
- **Diabetes.**
- **Fibromyalgia.**
- **Gastrointestinal diseases.**
- **Hay fever.**
- **Heart disease.**
- **Obesity.**
- **Periodontitis.**

Got your attention? Good.

Chronic inflammation is inflammation that takes place in the body over long periods of time. While scientists aren't sure whether inflammation causes these diseases or is the result of these diseases, inflammation has been linked to all of the diseases in the above list and more.

A poor diet is one of the leading causes of chronic inflammation. You already knew this, because everyone knows that eating processed foods and foods that are high in bad fats is bad for your health. You just didn't know why. One of the biggest reasons these foods are bad for you is their tendency to cause inflammation once they enter the body. You probably won't notice the inflammation when it's minor. It isn't until it build up to a crisis point that it reveals itself—usually in the form of a disease or illness.

The good news is there are a number of things you can do now to reduce inflammation in the body before it becomes a bigger problem. Here are some of the things you can do to preemptively strike and cut down on inflammation:

- **Cut back on your sugar intake.**
- **Eat a healthy diet that contains small amounts of good fats.**
- **Eat more berries and cruciferous vegetables.**
- **Eat more omega-3 rich fish.**
- **Eat more turmeric.**
- **Eliminate partially hydrogenated fats from your diet.**
- **Eliminate trans fats from your diet.**

- **Exercise regularly.**
- **Keep the amount of dairy you eat to a minimum.**
- **Keep the amount of wheat (and gluten) you eat to a minimum.**
- **Lose weight (if you're overweight).**
- **Stay away from artificial sweeteners.**
- **Stop drinking.**
- **Stop eating fast food.**
- **Stop eating fried food.**
- **Stop eating junk food.**
- **Stop eating processed foods.**
- **Stop smoking.**
- **Switch to pastured animal meat.**

In addition to the items on the above list, you can add coconut oil to your diet—or, better yet, use it to replace other vegetable oils known to cause inflammation. Partially-hydrogenated oils contain trans fats that are especially bad and should be avoided at all costs, but even the oils that are said to be "heart-healthy" can cause inflammation as they go rancid.

There's no shortage of studies showing coconut oil to be an effective anti-inflammatory. Virgin coconut oil has been shown in studies to have strong anti-inflammatory properties (19) and MCTs, which coconut oil is packed with, are known to enhance the inflammatory immune response (20). Coconut oil has been proven to have anti-inflammatory, analgesic and antipyretic properties (21).

Coconut oil may be one of the better foods you can add to your diet to help knock out inflammation. If you want to preemptively strike against inflammation or you suspect you have health problems that are due to inflammation, consult with your primary health care provider to see if coconut oil is a viable option. If it is, it's worth a shot because of the health benefits associated with it, not the least of which is its ability to fight inflammation.

Coconut Oil for Allergy Relief

Allergies come in a number of forms. Food allergies and airborne allergies are two of the most common, and both can be helped through use of coconut oil.

Dairy allergies are one of the most common food allergies around. While some people know they're allergic because the reaction is immediate and severe, others suffer dairy allergies for years without realizing the side effects they're suffering is due to dairy consumption.

Here are some of the symptoms of dairy allergies:

- **Bloating.**
- **Bloody stools.**
- **Brain fog.**
- **Burping.**
- **Colic.**
- **Congestion.**
- **Coughing.**
- **Cramping.**
- **Diarrhea.**
- **Fatigue.**
- **Flushing.**
- **Gas.**
- **Hives.**
- **Itchy skin.**
- **Problems breathing.**
- **Rashes.**
- **Upset stomach.**

- **Vomiting.**
- **Watery eyes.**

An allergic reaction to dairy starts when the body has an immune system response to a dairy product. The dairy food is seen as a foreign invader and the body treats it as such, attacking it and seeking to eliminate it from the body. The reaction to dairy can be severe, even to the point where it's life threatening.

Coconut oil and coconut milk (which contains coconut oil) can be used to replace dairy in your diet. People who are allergic to dairy products are more often than not able to process and digest coconut oil and coconut milk. If you suspect you're suffering from mild dairy allergies, you can switch to coconut products to see if the symptoms subside. If they do, you'll know you were mildly allergic to the dairy. When I made the switch in my household, my husband and both of my children immediately saw relief from their chronically congested sinuses.

Never attempt to use coconut oil (or milk) to treat a severe allergic response to dairy. They're good replacements, but aren't going to do much good during a severe allergic reaction to dairy. Seek immediate medical attention if you're having a severe allergic reaction.

The symptoms of allergies come about due to inflammation. The body senses there's something wrong and calls in the troops. The troops attack and inflammation occurs as a result. That's right, allergy symptoms are due to the same inflammation that coconut has been shown to knock down. If you're having a bad allergic reaction, coconut oil probably isn't going to do much. You need to get to a doctor as soon as possible. On the other hand, you may be able to help ease up minor allergies without having to go to the doctor. There's no shortage of people who claim to have eliminated their allergies through judicious use of coconut oil.

Allergies like hay fever (and a number of other allergies) can be alleviated by using coconut oil to boost the body's immune system. There are people who claim regular consumption of coconut oil has all but eliminated their airborne allergies. Most of the symptoms you suffer due to allergies are because your body is attacking the allergen and treating it like a dangerous foreign substance. During allergy season, your body is undergoing a constant "attack" from substances it sees as harmful. This constant battle can lead to the immune system wearing down and becoming more susceptible to illnesses and ailments.

You can consume coconut oil regularly to give your immune system a much-needed boost. This will help your body by keeping your immune system strong.

Yet another way coconut oil can help allergies is to dip your finger in it and spread it around the inside and outside of your nostrils. This will help prevent the lining of your nose from coming in contact with the pollen or whatever it is that's causing the irritation by catching the pollen before it gets inside. I was dubious when a friend told me to try this technique, but now I swear by it in the Spring and early Summer, when pollen is at its worst.

Coconut oil can help prevent allergies in a less obvious way. Studies have shown that asthma and allergic disorders may be tied to childhood use of antibiotics (22). It may be too late for you, but using coconut oil to treat minor bacterial and fungal infections naturally may help your children over the long run. I wish my mother would have had this information when I was a child. I may not have spent years suffering before I discovered coconut oil.

Enhance Nutrient Uptake with Coconut Oil

Fat-soluble nutrients are nutrients you eat that have to be digested with fat. Your body only needs small amounts of these nutrients to stay healthy because it stores them in the liver and in your body fat when it gets extra. Consuming fat-soluble vitamins in excess is dangerous, so be careful what vitamins you supplement your diet with. As long as you're eating a healthy and balanced diet, you probably don't need to supplement your diet with fat-soluble vitamins.

The fat-soluble vitamins your body needs are vitamins A, D, E and K.

If you're on a low-fat diet, your body may not be able to absorb enough of these nutrients to stay healthy. A study published in the online *Molecular Nutrition & Food Research* in June 2012 revealed that subjects fed salads with fatty oils in them absorbed more nutrients when they upped the amount of fat being added to their salads (22). What this means is eating a salad with low- or no-fat dressing may actually be worse for you than eating a salad with a fatty oil like coconut oil drizzled on it.

Instead of avoiding all fats, the better option is to include healthy fats healthy fats in your diet in small amounts—and coconut oil is one of those fats. At least some healthy fat should be consumed with every meal. Without it, fat-soluble vitamins will pass through your system without ever being used. It doesn't take a lot of fat, but you need at least a little to get the most from your meal. Coconut oil has proven itself to be one of the better fats when it comes to nutrient absorption. In a study where coconut oil was compared to safflower oil, coconut oil aided absorption of fat-soluble nutrients from tomatoes at a higher level than safflower oil (23). In another study, coconut oil beat out both canola and safflower oil (24).

The human body needs small amounts of good fat to survive and there's rarely good reason to deprive it of the fat it needs. What good is a low-fat diet if it sacrifices the health of the person on it because they aren't getting the most out of the meals they eat? That's not to say you should go out and start eating all the fat you can stuff in your face. The key is to eat good fats that help you absorb nutrients.

The reason coconut oil stands head and shoulders above most other oils in this department is the high levels of MCTs found in the oil.

The human digestive system has a tough time digesting the LCTs in other oils. The pancreas has to make special enzymes to digest LCTs. As we get older, our bodies produce less of these enzymes, which means even slower digestion of LCTs. The MCTs in coconut oil don't require this enzyme to be digested, so they're processed quickly and sent to the liver. This propensity for quick digestion gives them the edge because they're able to help the body take in fat-soluble nutrients at a brisk pace.

This hasn't gone unnoticed by the medical community.

MCTs have seen use to help treat people with digestive and malabsorption issues. They deliver nourishment in a convenient package that's easy to digest and boosts absorption of other nutrients at the same time.

The MCTs in coconut oil are beneficial to most people, but are especially beneficial for those who struggle to digest the longer fatty acid chains found in other oils. Coconut oil has been used to aid digestion and ease symptoms in those with the following conditions:

- **Constipation.**
- **Inflammatory bowel disease (IBD).** Studies have shown MCTs to be effective in decreasing inflammation in the gut (25).
- **Irritable bowel syndrome (IBS).** IBS isn't as bad as IBD, but it can still be difficult to deal with. The cause isn't clear, but may be linked to unhealthy bacteria, which coconut oil can help eliminate.
- **Malabsorption.**
- **Pancreatitis.** The pancreas produces enzymes used to digest LCTs. When you eat a diet high in long-chain fatty acids, there's a heavy load placed on your pancreas. The MCTs in coconut oil don't require the same enzymes as LCTs, so switching to coconut oil can ease the load on your pancreas.
- **Patients with severe digestive problems.**
- **Patients with gall bladder problems.** Gall bladder removal can result in patients having trouble digesting LCTs. The MCTs in coconut oil are much easier for a patient without a gall bladder to handle.

- **Premature infants with underdeveloped digestive systems.**
- **Stomach ulcers.**
- **Sufferers of Crohn's disease.** A number of people claim eating coconut macaroons, which are high in coconut oil has helped ease the effects of Crohn's disease.
- **Ulcerative colitis.**

MCTs are added to feeding formulas for the sick and for infants in hospitals because they're easy to digest and they up nutrient intake. Premature infants often have digestive issues and MCTs are included as part of their formula because of their ease of digestion.

In addition to being easy to digest, coconut oil gives your immune system a boost and helps eliminate bad bacteria in your gut. It's even effective against bacteria that have built up immunity to antibiotics and modern medicines.

There's no reason you can't get the same effect at home.

See the chapter titled "Adding Coconut Oil to Your Diet" at the end of this book for ideas on how you can add coconut oil to your diet. You can cook with it, add it to smoothies and other drinks or you can take it as a supplement before your meal. No matter how it's taken, the MCTs in coconut oil will go to work making sure you get the most from your food.

Give Breast Milk a Healthy Boost

Human breast milk is the closest thing you're going to find to a perfect food. It's designed to provide infants with all the nutrients they need for the first year or two they're alive—or at least until they develop teeth and start to bite down.

The blend of nutrients contains everything an infant needs to thrive.

Lauric acid is one of the main ingredients in breast milk, along with a number of other MCTs with similar properties. If it weren't for lauric acid and the other fatty acids in breast milk, infants would be a lot more susceptible to disease.

The MCTs found in breast milk are easy on a newborn child's digestive system and are easily broken down into units of energy. Infants have sensitive digestive systems that are prone to problems as they mature. MCTs ease the load on the digestive system because of how easy they are for the body to synthesize. They also protect the baby from disease, infection and a number of other potentially deadly health issues.

The amount of MCTs found in breast milk varies from mother to mother. Just how healthy a mother's milk is depends on how healthy the mother is and what she puts into her body. Eating good foods full of vitamins and nutrients means the baby gets lots of vitamins and nutrients in its milk. Living an unhealthy lifestyle results in a mother passing unhealthy substances into her breast milk. Trans fats, drugs and other toxins can all be passed from a mother into her breast milk.

The mother's diet has a direct influence on the fatty acid content of the mother's milk. Consume large amounts of polyunsaturated fat and the breast milk will contain elevated levels of polyunsaturated fat. Consume coconut oil and the lauric acid level in the milk goes up. 2 to 3 tablespoons of coconut oil can more than double the amount of lauric acid found in breast milk for as long as 12 hours.

Lactating mothers can supplement their diets with 3 to 4 tablespoons of coconut oil a day to ensure their babies are getting the healthiest breast milk possible. Infants deserve the best possible start in life and breast milk high in lauric acid gives them that start.

The Candida Killer

Candida albicans is the bacteria that's the driving force behind a number of misdiagnosed health problems in the world today. An overgrowth of these bacteria, also known as a yeast infection, can cause all sorts of problems in the body.

Here are some of the more common symptoms associated with candida:

- **Aches and pains.**
- **ADD.**
- **ADHD.**
- **Allergies.**
- **Alopecia.**
- **Anorexia.**
- **Anxiety.**
- **Asthma.**
- **Athletes foot.**
- **Bad smells.**
- **Bloating.**
- **Brain fog.**
- **Bulimia.**
- **Colds.**
- **Confusion.**
- **Constipation.**
- **Coughing.**
- **Depression.**
- **Diarrhea.**
- **Digestive problems.**

- Eczema.
- Excess abdominal fat.
- Excessive sweating.
- Fatigue.
- Fibromyalgia.
- Fungal infections.
- Headaches.
- Heartburn.
- High blood pressure.
- Hypothyroidism.
- Impotence.
- Infections.
- Infertility.
- Intense sugar cravings.
- Irregular heartbeat.
- Irritability.
- Itching.
- Jock itch.
- Lack of sexual prowess.
- Low blood sugar.
- Lupus.
- Memory loss.
- Metabolic syndrome.
- Migraines.
- Mood swings.
- Numbness.
- OCD.
- Panic attacks.
- Psoriasis.

- **Rashes.**
- **Ringworm.**
- **Runny nose.**
- **Sinus problems.**
- **Sleep problems.**
- **Stuffy head.**
- **Vaginal discharge.**

A quick run-down of the problems on this list reveals many issues that can crop up that doctors will attempt to treat on their own without looking to see whether candida is to blame. Keep in mind that candida isn't the only cause of these problems and isn't always to blame, but it is the culprit often enough that it warrants a closer look, especially if you're suffering from multiple issues on the list—or any number of other issues that haven't been listed. This list isn't all-inclusive by any means.

The problem with treating the symptoms is that you completely ignore the cause. Treat one symptom and a new one may pop up somewhere else. Or two. Or three. Or four. Once you stop taking medication for the symptom you're treating, it can come back with a vengeance, leading your doctor to prescribe stronger medications. The medication causes other problems to crop up and you're soon ingesting a cocktail of medications that help line the pockets of drug manufacturers, but do little to solve your problems.

Even when it's known that candida is the cause of your woes, doctors will more often than not prescribe antibiotics that kill both the candida and good bacteria in your body. It's difficult to completely kill off a candida overgrowth because it can spread across pretty much your entire body.

Once the antibiotics are stopped, the candida comes back—and it can build up a resistance to the antibiotics. The next time around, the candida are harder to kill and the antibiotics aren't as effective.

Coconut oil combined with probiotic supplements may be an effective natural treatment for candida. The caprylic, capric and lauric acids found in coconut oil are able to kill candida cells by breaking through their cell walls.

When you first start taking coconut oil for candida, you're probably going to experience symptoms of a candida die-off as your body attempts to process and rid itself of all of the dead candida. Common symptoms include headaches, diarrhea and stomach cramps, and can range from mild to severe, depending on how pronounced the die-off is. You can ease the effects of the die-off by starting off only taking a tablespoon of coconut oil a day and then slowly ramping up to 3 to 4 tablespoons.

After taking coconut oil for a week or two, start taking a probiotic supplement. The healthy bacteria in the probiotic supplement should replace the candida as they die off and will crowd out any candida left alive.

Hemorrhoid Relief

Hemorrhoids, also known as piles, are swollen veins or groups of veins in or around the anus. While they aren't life-threatening, they can be painful and are the bane of many people's existence. They typically worsen over time, so it's important to get hemorrhoids treated when they first pop up.

Hemorrhoids can occur for the following reasons:

- **Frequent bouts of diarrhea.**
- **Hard stools.**
- **Large stools.**
- **Rough stools.**
- **Obesity.**
- **Old age.**
- **Pregnancy.**
- **Sitting on the toilet for extended periods of time.**
- **Straining while defecating.**

Some people are more prone to hemorrhoids than others, but most people suffer from at least one hemorrhoid over the course of their life. Other people are more susceptible to hemorrhoids and are seemingly constantly afflicted.

If you've ever suffered the itching, bleeding and pain associated with hemorrhoids, you've undoubtedly wanted relief . . . and fast! The itching and burning is a constant reminder that something isn't right down there and it can drive you up a wall. When you have a hemorrhoid that's acting up, sometimes it's all you can think about. You spend your waking hours suffering, hoping for relief.

There are a number of people who claim to have used coconut oil to cure hemorrhoids. There aren't any scientific evidence to back this claim up, but it bears mention because of the large number of people claiming it works.

Where coconut oil really comes into its own is as a means of relieving the itching and burning associated with hemorrhoids. You may still have to get your hemorrhoids treated and/or removed by a doctor, but coconut oil can provide at least some level of relief in the interim.

To use coconut oil to provide hemorrhoid relief, apply it topically to the affected area 3 to 5 times a day for a week. Every time you have a bowel movement, wipe the affected area clean and reapply a fresh coating of coconut oil. The itching and burning should ease up rather quickly. If those who say it works to shrink hemorrhoids are correct, you may see your hemorrhoids start to clear up within a couple days.

Health Problems? Give Your Thyroid a Boost

Have you thought about your thyroid lately?

Most people haven't. Most people have heard of their thyroid gland, but couldn't tell you where it's located in their body, let alone what it's there for. Well, I've got news for you. It's high time you started paying closer attention to your thyroid.

The next time you're in your doctor's office, ask him or her what the thyroid gland does. When they respond that it's "responsible for metabolism," ask them to elaborate and watch them squirm. I've yet to find a doctor who doesn't specialize in thyroid problems that is able to explain thyroid function accurately.

What I'm about to teach you is more than many doctors know about the thyroid and it could be the cause of many of your health problems. If you're suffering from health problems and are having trouble figuring out the cause, an underactive thyroid may be the reason.

Your thyroid gland is located underneath your Adam's apple on your neck. It isn't obvious and you probably would never notice it . . . Unless you have a problem that causes it to swell. The thyroid gland has one job, and that's to produce thyroid hormones. It's controlled by the pituitary gland, which tells it when to turn production of thyroid hormones off and on. The pituitary and thyroid glands work hand-in-hand to ensure the body has the right amount of thyroid hormones. The thyroid can't sense when the body needs more or less hormones and is unable to regulate thyroid hormone levels by itself.

The pituitary gland monitors thyroid hormone levels in the body (along with other hormone levels) and releases a hormone called TSH (thyroid stimulation hormone) that tells the thyroid it needs to ramp up production. When TSH levels are high, this is indicative that there isn't enough thyroid hormone in the body. When TSH levels are low, the body has higher levels of thyroid hormones.

Thyroid hormones are tied into your body's metabolism.

They regulate how fast your metabolism runs, how much energy your body burns and how fast it burns it. People with a high metabolism burn more energy and those with a low metabolism burn less energy. This is the reason why some people are able to eat like they have a hollow leg and not gain weight, while all others have to do is look at fattening food and they start packing on the pounds.

Thyroid hormones act upon almost every cell in the body. They increase and decrease your heart rate, they tell your body how fast to use oxygen and food to produce energy and they stimulate red blood cell production. They also stimulate the production of other hormones that are responsible for all sorts of processes in the body.

Problems abound when the thyroid gland is overactive (hyperthyroidism) or underactive (hypothyroidism). It isn't uncommon for those with thyroid issues to go undiagnosed for years, until the symptoms get bad enough they can't be ignored.

The following symptoms are associated with thyroid gland issues:

- **Aches and pains.**
- **Chills.**
- **Cold feet.**
- **Cold hands.**
- **Fatigue.**
- **Hair loss.**
- **Headaches.**
- **Insomnia.**
- **Loss of appetite.**
- **Low core body temperature.**
- **Mental fog.**
- **Rapid heartbeat.**
- **Tinnitus.**
- **Uncontrollable weight gain.**
- **Vertigo.**

Hypothyroidism is believed to be reaching epidemic proportions.

A study in which 25,862 people in Colorado were tested for thyroid dysfunction appears to confirm this suspicion. 9.5 percent of the people tested showed elevated TSH level. Surprisingly, 6 percent were taking thyroid hormones intended to regulate thyroid activity (26). If these numbers hold true across the entire United States, and there's no reason to believe they don't, there are nearly 30 million Americans who are suffering from hypothyroidism, many of whom haven't yet been diagnosed.

Further compounding the problem is the fact that some leading experts have gone on record as stating smaller imbalances in the thyroid that don't show up in TSH level testing can still cause problems. The number of people who are suffering from imbalances that are undetectable is unknown, but if consumption of soy oil and other oils high in unsaturated fats is to blame, the numbers could be astronomically high.

Thyroid problems, especially those associated with an underactive thyroid, are thought by many to be a result of our increased consumption of unsaturated fats and oils. Unsaturated oil depresses thyroid function, while saturated fats help ward off the effects of hypothyroidism. In an experiment published in the Online Journal of Health and Allied Sciences, rabbits fed a diet of coconut oil for 12 weeks gained less weight and had decreased levels of TSH in their blood, which is indicative of healthy thyroid function. Rabbits fed soybean oil showed increased TSH levels and gained more weight than the rabbits fed coconut oil (27).

While medication may be necessary in the short-term to treat thyroid problems, it does nothing to treat the underlying issue that's causing the low thyroid activity. The thyroid drugs being prescribed don't restore balance in the body and make the thyroid function properly. Most of them just replace the thyroid hormones the body is lacking.

Restoring proper thyroid function could be as simple as making the switch from soybean-based oils to coconut oil in your daily diet and avoiding foods that contain vegetable oils. Some people have seen improvements by adding 2 to

3 tablespoons of coconut oil to their diet as a supplement. Other foods that can be cut from the diet in order to improve thyroid health are all forms of sugar, refined grains, alcohol, caffeine and hydrogenated and partially-hydrogenated oils.

Add in a healthy exercise regime and some people may be able to get their thyroid hormones back in balance enough to kick thyroid drugs to the curb. Never stop using thyroid drugs on your own. Be sure to consult your doctor if you plan on trying to regulate your thyroid gland through diet and exercise. There may be underlying concerns you aren't aware of.

Can Coconut Oil Help You Lose Weight?

For years, we've been told to cut back on fats in our diet in order to lose weight. During this time, obesity rates have skyrocketed to somewhere in the range of 20% to 35%, depending on what area of the country you live in. Obesity rates have roughly doubled in the last 25 years and low-fat diets are largely failing to regulate weight gain.

Eliminating fat from your diet often doesn't help promote weight loss because it leaves the person on the diet feeling tired and hungry all the time. Instead of eating fat, the person over-eats carbs, which are even more likely to be stored as body fat. No matter how many carbs you eat, you still end up feeling hungry and unsatisfied. Lipids are the means through which the body determines whether it's satiated or not. A diet devoid of lipids doesn't provide the body with the fat it needs to feel satiated and leaves you feeling unsatisfied and famished.

When you hear people on a diet complain about how hungry they are, chances are they're on a low-fat diet—and there's a good chance they aren't going to be able to stick to it. Being hungry all the time wears you down and eventually you give in to your urges.

Studies are now revealing that it isn't the amount of fat being consumed inasmuch as it's the type of fat being consumed that packs on the pounds. Saturated fats have been the primary fat consumed by man for thousands of years, so it stands to reason the human body has adapted to being able to efficiently process these fats. Polyunsaturated fats were only found in foods in small amounts until recent years, so it stands to reason the human body is only capable of processing them in small amounts. Current dietary logic flips thousands of years of evolution on its head. Polyunsaturated fats are recommended over saturated fats even though humans have traditionally consumed a diet high in saturated fat from meat, eggs and dairy.

Coconut oil helps promote weight loss in the following ways:

- **It destroys bad bacteria like candida, which can promote weight gain.**
- **It has no trans fat.**
- **It makes you feel satiated for longer after eating.**
- **It prevents blood glucose fluctuations.**
- **It reduces abdominal fat.**
- **It slows down digestion.**
- **It speeds up metabolism.**
- **The fats in coconut oil are less likely to be stored as body fat than other types of fat.**

The MCFAs in coconut oil are more easily converted to energy and are less prone to being stored as body fat because of the way they're processed by the body. The LCFAs found in unsaturated oils are put out into the bloodstream, where they're more likely to be processed into body fat. MCFAs aren't circulated through the body and only enter the bloodstream for a short trip up through the portal vein. They're burned as fuel by the liver before the body has a chance to convert them to body fat.

Coconut oil boosts your metabolism and has been shown to reduce obesity. A clinical trial on 40 women between 20 and 40 years of age showed coconut oil to reduce body mass and abdominal obesity when their diet was supplement with 30mL of oil a day (7). Abdominal fat is considered one of the worst types of fat and is thought to be a precursor to other more serious health issues.

Medium-chain triglycerides have been shown to induce thermogenesis to a greater extent than long-chain triglycerides (28). They have been shown to aid in the prevention of obesity by speeding up the oxidation of fat and reducing upper body adipose tissue (29). One study showed a 12% increase in metabolic rate over the 6 hour period following consumption of MCTs (30). The propensity of coconut oil to act as a metabolism booster makes it a much safer alternative to diet pills packed full of caffeine and other stimulants that artificially boost metabolism.

When MCTs are used to replace LCTs in the diet, good things begin to happen. The body stores less fat because there are less LCTs available in the bloodstream for it to store. Instead of lowering overall fat consumption, try replacing vegetable oils laden with LCTs with coconut oil, which is full of MCTs. Your body won't store fat if it isn't present in the bloodstream, and MCT's largely eliminate fat from the bloodstream.

We briefly mentioned weight gain as one of the symptoms of hypothyroidism in the last chapter, but it bears mention again. A low-functioning thyroid can slow down metabolism and cause weight gain, *even when caloric intake remains the same.* People suffering rapid weight gain seemingly out of nowhere should get checked for hypothyroidism, especially if the weight gain is accompanied by other symptoms indicative of hypothyroidism.

Consuming coconut oil on its own probably isn't going to help you lose much weight. It may help you reduce waist size and abdominal fat, but if weight loss is your ultimate goal, you're going to need to up the ante. Replace other vegetable oils with coconut oil and reduce your carbohydrate and refined sugar consumption, and you'll probably start shedding those extra pounds.

It isn't the amount of fat that people consume that makes them fat. It's the type. Coconut oil consumed in moderation is good for most people and can be part of a healthy diet. Low-fat diets are hard to stick to because they leave you feeling hungry all the time. Adding saturated fat to your diet in the form of coconut oil has been shown to boost metabolism and is believed to promote weight loss.

The Healthy Energy Drink

In this day and age, it seems like we're always on the run. With all the responsibilities we have, it isn't uncommon to spend weeks on end running around from the beginning of the day to the end. After a while, we begin to wear down and need an energy boost to get us through the day.

Energy drink companies know this and sell expensive drinks guaranteed to give people the boost they need to make it through the day. What most people don't realize is they could end up paying a steep cost for that boost, especially if they're consuming energy drinks daily.

The ingredients found in most energy drinks leave a lot to be desired. Here are some of the more common ingredients and the dangers associated with them:

- **Ephedra or ephedrine.** This powerful stimulant, commonly found in energy drinks designed to help you lose weight, can cause a dangerous spike in your blood pressure (31). It's also used to manufacture meth. Probably not something you want in your body.
- **Taurine.** Taurine is an amino acid found in bull bile. It's manufactured by the body in small amounts, but the effect of larger amounts of taurine on the body isn't fully understood. You get all the taurine your body needs through your diet and adding more isn't necessary and may negatively impact your health.

- **Caffeine.** In small amounts, caffeine helps most people focus and stimulates the brain. In the amount found in energy drinks, it can leave you feeling jumpy and jittery. It's also addictive. If you crave your morning cup of coffee or a mid-day energy drink, the caffeine in the drink is a big part of the reason why.
- **Apartame.** If you're drinking sugar-free energy drinks, you may be drinking aspartame, which is thought by many to be one of the most dangerous substances allowed to be put in food. While food and health agencies largely say it's safe, a number of sources report it can cause adverse allergic reactions ranging from headaches to irregular heartbeat.
- **Sugar.** You wouldn't eat 16 teaspoons of sugar, would you? Energy drinks are some of the worst offenders when it comes to adding excess sugar to your diet. You may be adding as much as 80g of sugar is one fell swoop, which is roughly equivalent to 16 teaspoons of sugar. Yuck.

I've seen first-hand the effects of drinking too many energy drinks.

I worked with a man who drank 2 to 3 energy drinks a day. He'd start the workday with one in his hand and would finish the day by drinking another. He'd sometimes have one at lunch if he was really feeling worn down. When I first met this guy, he seemed like a normal person. Over the course of a year, I watched him slowly but surely become sicker and sicker.

As things progressed, he would go into mental lapses where he didn't know where he was and you couldn't talk to him because all he did was stare straight ahead. At first the mental lapses were sort of funny and people joked around about them. After a while, they got so bad he had to be hospitalized. One day at work, I was talking to him and he just sort of faded out. He went from being completely aware of his surroundings to being unable to hold a coherent conversation. He wasn't unconscious, but he wasn't responsive either. I walked him to the nearest break area, where he sat down and struggled to regain focus.

He ended up going to the doctor's office that day, at which time he was diagnosed with an irregular heartbeat, but the doctors weren't able to figure out why he'd faded out the way he had. After it happened a time or two more, someone suggested to him that it could be the energy drinks. He was dubious, but stopped drinking them just to see.

While there's no proof the drinks were to blame, there were no more episodes after he quit drinking them. He went back to leading a normal life and as far as I know hasn't had another lapse into semi-consciousness. Seeing the damage first-hand was enough to get me to swear off energy drinks for good.

The good news is there's a much safer alternative.

Coconut oil provides you with a quick and all-natural energy boost shortly after you consume it. It digests quickly and is sent straight to your liver where it's converted to energy in no time flat. If you're feeling rundown, a tablespoon or two of coconut oil may be all you need to perk up a bit.

I know what you're thinking, and I'm right there with you.

There's no caffeine in coconut oil. If you want to add a little caffeine, do so in the form of coffee. Coffee tastes great when you stir a tablespoon or two of coconut oil into it. The amount of caffeine in a cup of coffee won't make you jittery unless you're sensitive to caffeine and you don't get all the other potentially dangerous additives. You also don't get the mad rush of sugar that'll leave you feeling worn down and burnt out in no time at all.

All-Natural Skin Care

Skin problems rank amongst the most embarrassing problems a person can have, especially if they're in a highly visible area. Most skin problems aren't debilitating inasmuch as they're embarrassing and are a constant reminder that we're less than perfect. Smooth, silky skin is a hard to reach target that eludes most people. Rare is the person with perfect skin from top to bottom.

Acne, psoriasis, dermatitis, dry skin, wrinkles, etc. You name it; coconut oil can probably help. It's as close as you can get to a one-stop natural solution to all of your skin problems.

All those expensive products you've been using are drying out your skin and making things worse. The harsh astringents, chemical cleansers and synthetic scents found in many commercial "skin care" products may leave your skin feeling soft and smelling good in the short term, but they end up doing more harm than good over the long term.

Propylene glycol is one such chemical. It's a byproduct of petroleum refining that is used in antifreeze, as a solvent and as an emulsifier. It's found in toothpaste, skin care products and even some processed foods and drinks. There are a number of studies that show propylene glycol to be a mild dermal irritant (32), but there are no studies showing the long-term effects of applying small amounts of propylene glycol to the skin. You wouldn't rub antifreeze into your arms and face, would you? I don't recommend using products containing this chemical compound, especially since there's a safer alternative.

Coconut oil gets to the root of your skin problems and attempts to eliminate them naturally. The same properties that make coconut oil good for you on the inside of your body make it a good choice to apply topically. It has the following properties that are beneficial to your skin:

- **All-natural.**
- **Antibacterial.**
- **Anti-inflammatory.**
- **Antimicrobial.**
- **Antiseptic.**
- **Antioxidant.**
- **Emollient.**
- **Fights the effects of aging.**
- **Healing.**
- **Moisturizing.**
- **Nourishing.**
- **Wards off infection.**

Coconut oil has been used by those seeking a natural remedy for the following issues:

- **Acne.**
- **Chapped skin.**
- **Dermatitis.**
- **Diaper rash.**
- **Dry skin.**
- **Eczema.**
- **Fungal infections.**

- **Irritated skin.**
- **Psoriasis.**
- **Rashes.**
- **Rosacea.**
- **Stretch marks.**
- **Wrinkles.**

These aren't just home remedies based on anecdotal evidence. There are a number of scientific studies that show coconut oil is a great choice for skin care:

- A 2008 study by the Skin and Cancer Foundation in the Philippines found that coconut oil may be an effective treatment for atopic dermatitis (33).
- A 2009 UC San Diego study found that lauric acid, which is found in abundance in coconut oil, is a potential alternative therapy for acne vulgaris (34).
- A 2004 study by the Department of Dermatology at the Makati Medical Center in the Philippines concluded that coconut oil is "effective and safe" when used as a skin moisturizer (35).

Virgin coconut oil has a low melting point (76 degrees F) and the MCTs in the oil are easily absorbed deep within the skin. The MCTs stay in liquid form once they enter your body and are so small they aren't likely to clog up your pores. Never use partially-hydrogenated coconut oil for skin care (or for anything else, for that matter) because it has a much higher melting point and can solidify in your pores, clogging them up.

Your skin cells are able to utilize the MCTs in coconut oil to promote healing and to generate new skin cells. Rubbing coconut oil into your skin ensures your body has a readily available source of nutrition and energy for the skin when it needs it. This regenerative property of coconut oil makes it a great serum to reverse the effects of aging and to prevent new wrinkles from forming.

Coconut oil has been shown to promote healing when it's applied to wounds. One study found that wounds treated with virgin coconut oil heal at a significantly faster rate than untreated wounds (36).

To use coconut oil for skin care, apply it topically a couple times a day. If the skin condition worsens or doesn't start to get better after a day or two, discontinue use and contact your physician immediately. Coconut oil can be used to heal dry and damaged skin. It can also be used as a preventative measure to prevent the damage from happening in the first place.

The All-Natural Athlete's Foot Cure

Athlete's foot (and other fungal infections) can be tough to deal with. The itching, cracking and burning make you miserable, not to mention the fact that you can't wear flip flops or sandals because your feet look like they were attacked by a wolverine. Summer time is rough because when you do venture to the pool, you get sideways glances from everyone that sees the sad shape your feet are in.

Over-the-counter athlete's foot medications rarely work and prescription medications cost a small fortune and aren't much better. If you're lucky, they ease the irritation enough to make it tolerable. They may even make it go away for a while, but you know as soon as you stop medicating, the fungus will be back.

If you've been struggling with athlete's foot, I have good news for you. Coconut oil has strong anti-fungal properties and can help you finally get rid of that foot fungus that's been driving you nuts.

When it comes to using coconut oil to get rid of athlete's foot, a two-pronged approach seems to works best. If you aren't already doing so, try adding a couple teaspoons of coconut oil to your diet. For minor fungal infections, this may be all that's required to clear things up. If the infection doesn't start to clear up in a couple days, it's time to kick things into high gear.

Apply a thick coating of coconut oil to the infected area first thing in the morning when you wake up. Try to keep it on for as long as you can before putting your sock on. Midday, apply another coating. Then apply it again in the evening. Before long, your athlete's foot should start clearing up. The first time I tried this it took about five days for my feet to clear up. After the infection started to clear up, I cut it back to a couple times a day because I was tired of having to apply it at work. It continued to clear and hasn't come back since.

Continue consuming coconut oil as part of your diet and monitor your feet. If you see signs of an infection, apply coconut oil to the irritated area until the infection goes away.

Cloth Diapers and Diaper Rash

Cloth diapers are great for the environment and can save you a lot of money, especially if you have multiple children in diapers at the same time. The savings can really add up over the 2 to 4 years your child is in diapers.

Diaper rash due to candida yeast can be a big problem with cloth diapers and it can be a tough one to get rid of because there's the chance of reinfection when diapers are reused. Just when it looks like the problem is under control, it can pop back up. Yeast infections are common after a child takes a course of antibiotics to treat another issue because it kills both good and bad bacteria. This can allow the yeast to gain a foothold and crowd out healthy bacteria.

The antifungal properties of coconut oil make it a good choice for diaper rash due to yeast (37). The coconut oil contains a number of fatty acids that are able to attack and kill a candida infection.

To treat diaper rash due to yeast, both the child and the items that touch the infected area have to be treated to rid them of yeast. Treating the baby is easy. Rub coconut oil on the affected area each time the child's diaper is changed. If the rash gets worse, discontinue use. If the rash starts to heal, keep using the coconut oil as diaper cream until the rash is gone.

Candida can live outside the body and reinfect an infant when a diaper is reused at a later time. Wash clothes, diapers, changing pads, wipes and anything else that comes in contact with the child with oxygenated bleach after each use. It may be necessary to make the switch to disposable diapers until the yeast infection is cured.

You can make an even more effective diaper rash cream by adding a tablespoon of zinc oxide to a cup of melted coconut oil and blending it with a stick blender as it solidifies. This cream can be used as an alternative to commercial diaper rash creams that contain a lot of unnecessary additives. If you use this cream, use a disposable diaper liner because the zinc can build up on the diaper and create a barrier that repels moisture instead of absorbing it.

If your child has a persistent diaper rash, consult with your health care provider before attempting to use coconut oil to treat it. While there's a good chance a persistent rash is yeast, there's always the possibility it could be something else that needs immediate medical attention.

Eliminate Acne

Acne is the number one most common skin problem afflicting people today. Some people are lucky and only have to deal with it during their teenage years, while others battle acne their entire lives.

Acne is caused by infections in the sebum glands, which are the glands in your skin that secrete oil to keep your skin from drying out and cracking. Bacteria and gunk builds up in the gland and it becomes inflamed and irritated.

The lauric acid in coconut oil has been shown to combat acne (38).

It can be used to help eliminate cystic acne and most other acne types. All you have to do is spread it on the area where the acne is present and let it go to work. The anti-inflammatory properties of the coconut oil will help relieve the swelling and associated pain and the antibacterial and antifungal properties of the oil will attack the root cause of the acne and help prevent new breakouts.

It's especially important that you only use unrefined virgin coconut oil for acne relief because partially-hydrogenated oils have a higher melt point and can solidify after they enter your pores, causing more acne to form instead of helping your acne.

You can use coconut oil to pull impurities from your skin by rubbing it in and leaving it there for a half hour to 45 minutes. It will pull the toxins and impurities to the surface of your skin. Use a steaming hot washcloth to clean your face and you'll be good to go.

In addition to spreading coconut oil on the skin to help fight acne, taking it internally helps as well. In a review of existing literature, researchers concluded that gut microbes contribute to acne (39). Since coconut oil helps regulate harmful bacteria in the gut, it stands to reason it can attack acne from this angle as well.

Ditch the harsh astringents and chemical packed cleansers and heal your skin the natural, healthy way.

All-Natural Hair Care

With everything else coconut oil is good for, are you really surprised that it's also good for your hair?

In a study on the prevention of hair damage, coconut oil, mineral oil and sunflower oil were all tested and coconut oil was the only oil found to reduce protein loss from hair in both damaged and undamaged hair. The other two oils had a negligible effect on protein loss (40). Coconut oil has a natural affinity for the protein found in hair, which pulls the oil inside the holes in the cuticles of the hair. Once inside, coconut oil then repels water, keeping it from entering the hair and causing further damage.

Coconut oil has been shown to penetrate the shaft of the hair, while mineral oil largely fails to get inside. This natural affinity allows coconut oil to get deep inside the hair and studies show it prevents the hair from swelling with water (41).

Using coconut oil in your hair before you wash it goes a long way toward making sure water doesn't get inside your hair and cause damage during the wash process. You can clean excess dirt and grime out of your hair without having to worry about doing more damage to it. The more damaged your hair is, the more holes it's going to have through which water can enter. This makes adding coconut oil to your hair even more important when you have damaged hair. Add it to your hair, let it sit for 10 to 15 minutes and then rinse it out before washing and conditioning your hair.

Coconut oil has also shown itself to be a good hair detangler. A study published in the Journal of Cosmetic Science in 1999 found that coconut oil worked well to prevent combing damage in both chemically bleached and thermally damaged hair. It prevented the cuticles from lifting and catching on one another, which is one of the main causes of hair breakage when brushing and combing the hair (42).

Don't be misled by the literature out there indicating coconut oil is a good moisturizer. It doesn't add moisture to your hair, which is what a true moisturizer does. Instead, it strengthens the hair shaft and locks the moisture that's already in the hair inside.

Dandruff Control

A flake or two on a black shirt is something most people have had to deal with. It's a bit embarrassing, but nothing out of the ordinary. It doesn't really get disconcerting until dandruff starts to get out of control, leaving white flakes on everything you touch and wear.

I know how bad it can get. I used to have bad dandruff and no matter what I did, I wasn't able to get it under control. I couldn't wear dark colors because within minutes I'd look like I'd eaten a powdered donut and dropped crumbs all over my shirt. I tried the shampoos, which provided relief for a while and then stopped working, and a number of natural remedies, most of which didn't work at all.

It wasn't until I discovered coconut oil that I was able to find relief from my dandruff.

Dandruff is sometimes caused by the malassezia globosa fungus. This fungus loves oily scalp because it feeds off of your natural oils. The problem with malassezia globosa is it creates oleic acid as a byproduct of eating your scalp oils, which makes your skin shed off in small chunks.

If your ears perked up when you saw the word fungus in the previous paragraph, kudos, you've been paying close attention. Coconut oil is a natural fungicide that seeks and destroys fungal infections naturally.

All you have to do is rub coconut oil into your scalp and let it sit overnight and it will go to work killing off the fungus causing your dandruff. Massage the oil into your scalp and put a shower cap over your head so you don't get coconut oil everywhere. When you wake up in the morning, wash the coconut oil out of your hair and go about your daily business. When the evening comes around again, repeat the process. Continue treating your hair with coconut oil until your dandruff goes away.

Once you've got rid of the dandruff and have killed off the fungus, you can stop treating your hair with coconut oil every day. Once or twice a week should be all it takes to keep your hair free of flakes. You get the added bonus of coconut oil being great for your hair's health and you'll have shiny, lustrous hair as a result.

Oh No, Not Head Lice!

Rare is the family that makes it through elementary school without at least one infection of head lice. I used to dread the accusatory phone call from the school nurse, who would rudely call and tell me my kids have lice and need to be picked up and treated before they can return to school.

Contrary to what this nurse seemed to believe, head lice are not a result of living in unsanitary conditions. I kept my house as clean as the next mom with three kids (reasonably clean, with the occasional day where I just gave up) and my kids still caught it. Lice don't pick their victims by testing to see who's clean or not. They jump from head to head at school. All it takes is for your kid to brush against the hair of another kid with lice and, BOOM, you get that dreaded phone call. It makes no difference how clean your house or your kids are.

Having had three kids all in elementary school at once, I battled these persistent near-microscopic bugs multiple times. The first few times I went to war with lice I did so with the chemical shampoos sold in the store. To be honest with you, they worked just fine. The problem with these shampoos is they contain toxic chemicals that kill the lice. When I made the switch to all-natural products, I had to find something that worked on lice. I searched far and wide and finally came across a post on a forum somewhere talking about using coconut oil as a natural remedy for lice. It worked great, and I've been using it ever since.

Coconut oil mixed with anise oil has been shown to be a more effective alternative treatment than permethrin, which is an active ingredient used in some lice shampoos (43). This is good news because coconut oil is non-toxic and is actually good for your hair.

There are three steps required to get rid of lice:

1. **Treat the hair and scalp to kill the lice.**
2. **Comb the nits out of the hair.**
3. **Treat the home to get rid of lice.**

While these steps may sound simple, anyone who's dealt with a difficult infestation can attest to how hard it is to get rid of lice. Let's take a closer look at each of the three steps.

Step 1: Treating the Hair and Scalp

This is the easy part.

Coat the hair and scalp with a thick coating of coconut oil and place a shower cap over the hair. Leave the shower cap on for an hour or two. Remove it and rinse the coconut oil from the hair.

The coconut oil coats the bodies of the lice and suffocates them. It doesn't kill lice eggs or prevent reinfestation, so you have to repeat this treatment once a day for at least a week. This will kill any new lice that hatch after the hair has been treated. It'll also kill any lice that attempt to move into the hair from objects in your house.

Step 2: Comb Out the Nits

This is the step most people hate.

You have to get rid of the nits, which are lice eggs, and any remaining lice in the hair.

Use an extremely fine toothed comb to remove the nits by thoroughly combing the hair. Failure to get rid of the nits will result in more lice hatching and reinfesting the hair. Even if you've killed all the lice with coconut oil, leaving nits in the hair will result in new lice infesting the hair within a day or two. You can get combs specifically made for combing out nits at the drug store for a couple bucks.

To get all the nits, shampoo and condition the hair and separate it into small sections. Start as close as you can get to the scalp and comb each section of hair out to the end. Make sure you use a comb that has small teeth that are designed for nit removal. Using a regular comb will leave a lot of nits in the hair.

As you finish a section, wipe the nits off of the comb with a tissue and move on to the next section. Clip or rubber band each section as you finish with it, so you know it's been combed. Carefully work your way through the entire head of hair. Once you're done, scan each section of hair for any nits you may have missed and comb them out or pull them out with your fingernails.

Dispose of the comb after using it. You're going to want to use a new comb each time you comb out nits. Alternatively, you can boil or otherwise disinfect the comb, but they're cheap enough that it's best to just throw the comb away and use a new one.

Step 3: Treat the Home

Lice can live in bedding and clothing for quite some time and can be picked back up at a later time. To prevent this from happening, wash all bedding and clothing in water that's hotter than 140 degrees F. Alternatively, you can place items you don't want to wash with hot water in the freezer. This will kill all lice and nits.

Rinse and repeat steps1 through 3 until you've cleared up the lice. It's going to take tenacity, but stick with it and you can get rid of lice naturally without having to use harsh chemicals to kill the bugs.

Don't forget to tell everyone your kids may have come in contact with while infested with lice. Sure, it can be a bit embarrassing, but you don't want your kids going to a friend's house and bringing lice back home. Treating your family and house for lice is bad enough the first time around. You don't want to have to repeat it a week or two down the road!

Diabetes

Nearly 30 million people in the United States alone have diabetes, and that number is expected to double in the next ten years. According to the Center for Disease Control, nearly 80 million Americans are pre-diabetic, which means they're on the cusp of contracting diabetes. Worldwide, a staggering 250 million people are estimated to have diabetes.

Type 2 diabetes, the most common type of diabetes, occurs when the body either doesn't produce the insulin it needs to regulate blood sugar or the insulin is there, but the cells don't use it. Insulin is used by the body to regulate glucose, or blood sugar, and without it, glucose begins to build up in the blood. Insulin resistance is a precursor to diabetes. As the body becomes more resistant to insulin, it isn't able to process glucose in the blood.

Having excess glucose in the blood for extended periods of time can cause all sorts of health problems. When you're diabetic, your body doesn't get the nourishment and energy it needs from the food you eat, which can result in you feeling hungry all the time. You'll feel run down no matter how much you eat because your body isn't able to properly process the food you're eating into energy units the body can use.

The following are some of the complications that can arise from diabetes:

- **Blurry vision.**
- **Dizziness.**

- Fatigue.
- Frequent urination.
- Gum disease.
- Hearing loss.
- Heart disease.
- High blood pressure.
- Hunger.
- Infections.
- Irritability.
- Kidney disease.
- Nerve damage.
- Numbness in the extremities.
- Open sores that don't heal.
- Skin infections.
- Stroke.
- Weight loss.

While the exact cause of diabetes and what sets it off in some people and not others isn't fully understood, there are a handful of risk factors that place people at higher risk of contracting the disease. Age, race and genetics all play a role, as do controllable factors like weight, how active you are and your diet. Eating bad fats and overconsumption of sugar leads to weight gain, which drastically ups your odds of triggering the onset of diabetes.

Diabetes typically progresses over time.

At first, most people are able to regulate it by eating a healthy diet and taking oral medication. As it progresses, a number of people have to start injecting themselves with insulin in order to ensure the body is getting the insulin it needs.

For many years, it was thought that once you contracted diabetes, it was irreversible. It was believed that, at best, you could hope to stall or slow the progression of the disease. It's now known that drastic changes in lifestyle and diet can reverse diabetes and get blood glucose levels back under control in some people. A 2011 study published in the journal *Diabetologia* showed that dramatic diet change can reverse the effects of diabetes within 8 weeks (44).

Replacing other vegetable oils with coconut oil may be a good choice for those who are diabetic or prediabetic. Wait a minute, you're probably saying. Aren't saturated fats bad for diabetics?

The answer isn't as simple as stating all saturated fats are bad and need to be avoided. There's evidence that seems to indicate coconut oil is a healthy choice when compared to other oils. A 2010 study published in the Indian Journal of Pharmacology revealed that coconut oil improves glucose tolerance while palm oil and ground nut oils impair glucose tolerance in rats with type 2 diabetes (45). Another study done by the University of Colorado determined that a diet containing MCTs increases insulin-mediated glucose metabolism in diabetic patients (46).

In addition to helping regulate glucose tolerance and metabolism, coconut oil provides your body with a ready source of energy. This quick energy boost provides your body the energy it desires a short time after consuming the oil, which can reduce hunger cravings associated with lack of energy. Instead of consuming refined carbohydrates which require insulin to process into energy, coconut oil knocks hunger out quickly and efficiently.

While more studies need to be done (and undoubtedly will), coconut oil looks to be a healthy dietary choice for diabetics due to the MCTs it contains. It helps regulate glucose tolerance, cuts down body fat and speeds up the body's metabolic rate while providing a quick energy boost without having to eat refined carbs.

Alzheimer's Disease and Coconut Oil

Alzheimer's disease is a form of dementia that generally sets in after 65 years of age, but has been known to start as early as 40 or 50. This incurable disease more often than not acts quickly. According to the Alzheimer's Association, those afflicted with this disease only live an average of 8 years from the time symptoms become apparent to others.

Symptoms of Alzheimer's disease include the following:

- **Confusion with placing names and faces.**
- **Constantly losing things.**
- **Forgetting how to do stuff that should be easy to do.**
- **Inability to remember recent occurrences.**
- **Inability to solve problems.**
- **Losing track of time or location.**
- **Memory loss.**
- **Mood swings or changes.**
- **Poor judgment.**
- **Problems talking.**
- **Problems writing.**
- **Social withdrawal.**

If you or a loved one is suffering from any of these symptoms, it's a good idea to get checked for Alzheimer's disease. It's important to note that, while these symptoms are sometimes indicative of the onset of Alzheimer's disease, they aren't exclusive to Alzheimer's disease and some may be part of the normal aging process.

The symptoms of Alzheimer's get worse over time. Sufferers may start with mild memory loss, but can eventually progress all the way to complete inability to function in any meaningful way.

While the exact cause of Alzheimer's disease isn't known, it's believed that it's caused by a number of factors combined. Oxidative damage due to lipid peroxidation is believed to be a contributing factor (47). Low-fat diets high in polyunsaturated fats prone to oxidation may be at least partially to blame for the rapid rise in Alzheimer's cases in recent years. Combine that with the aging of America's baby boomer generation and you have a problem that isn't going away any time soon. Currently there are more than 25 million people living with Alzheimer's disease worldwide. That number may increase to as high as 100 million people in the next 30 or so years.

This raises the question as to whether there's anything that can be done.

As of the writing of this book, millions of dollars have been poured into researching Alzheimer's disease, but modern medicine has largely failed to produce a cure. What researchers have determined is that a poor diet that's high in carbs and sugar and low in fats may be a precursor to Alzheimer's disease. An MIT Cambridge study concluded that excess carbohydrates in the diet combined with a deficiency in dietary fats and cholesterol "may lead to the development of Alzheimer's disease" (48).

Coconut oil contains high levels of dietary fats and increases the HDL cholesterol your brain needs to function properly. The saturated fats it contains aren't prone to oxidation and are more stable than unsaturated fats. Coconut oil may not be a cure for Alzheimer's, but it does help prevent some of the factors that are thought to cause it to set in.

Speaking of causative factors, there's mounting evidence that statin drugs may be contributing to Alzheimer's, or at least making the symptoms worse once Alzheimer's starts to set in. Researchers in a recent pilot study found that statin drugs "produce adverse effects on cognition in individuals with dementia" and showed that discontinuing use of statin drugs improved cognition (49). This is indicative that lowering cholesterol through use of drugs may limit the cholesterol the brain needs to function normally. More studies of the long-term effects of statin drugs on the brain are needed.

There are a handful of anecdotal stories floating around that appear to show coconut oil may be able to play a role in restoration of cognitive function in those who already have Alzheimer's disease. There's no scientific proof that coconut oil can cure (or at least ease the effects of) Alzheimer's disease, but stories of people who started taking coconut oil and saw almost instant improvement aren't all that uncommon.

I'll tell you this much. If I or a loved one was suffering from Alzheimer's disease, I'd stop at nothing to find something that at least slows this deadly disease down. While experimentation on coconut oil and Alzheimer's disease is in its infancy, that wouldn't stop me from trying it.

As with all treatment regimes, consult with a doctor or medical professional before making any changes to your diet or your medications.

Coconut Oil and Cancer

Let me begin this section by making one thing explicitly clear. Coconut oil is not a miracle cure for cancer. If you've been diagnosed with cancer, you need to consult with a medical professional as to the proper course of treatment for whatever cancer it is you've diagnosed with.

The interaction between coconut oil and various types of cancer is a complicated and inexact science. I've seen coconut oil touted online as a "cure" for cancer, which is a total misrepresentation of its capabilities. I can't in good conscience make this claim, as I don't think coconut oil alone is capable of treating cancer once it's got a foothold in the body.

It may be capable of slowing the growth of certain types of tumors, but the research into this phenomenon is in its infancy. An experiment comparing long-chain triglycerides (LCTs) with medium-chain triglycerides (MCTs) and their effect on weight loss and tumor growth in animals found that MCT's reduced both weight loss and tumor size in mice with adenocarcinoma of the colon (50). Another experiment determined that medium-chain triglycerides don't affect mammary tumorigenesis (51).

Where coconut oil really comes into its own is as a healthy alternative to oils that are full of trans fats, which have been linked to cancer. The saturated fats in coconut oil are much less likely to oxidize and form free radicals once they enter the body, making it a safer alternative to hydrogenated oils that are packed full of polyunsaturated fats that are prone to damage.

Experiments on animals have shown saturated fats to have little to no effect on tumor growth, while polyunsaturated fats cause tumors to increase in size at a faster clip. In an experiment done on rats, polyunsaturated fats were found to be responsible for higher tumor yields than saturated fats (52). Experiments in a laboratory setting at the University of Western Ontario showed a diet high in polyunsaturated fats and linoleic acid to promote the growth of mammary tumors in rats (53).

This is believed to be due to the linoleic content of polyunsaturated fat. Linoleic acid is not recognized by the body as a digestible fat and is unable to be processed once it enters the body. While it's unclear whether findings of lab tests on animals apply in the same manner to humans as they do lab rats, one thing's for certain. More research needs to be done into the connection between polyunsaturated fats, linoleic acid and cancer.

Until the verdict is in, I'm going to stick with coconut oil.

Watch What You Put In Your Mouth

Have you read the label on your toothpaste and mouthwash lately? If you're using a commercially sold toothpaste or mouthwash, you're more than likely bathing your teeth, gums and tongue in a chemical cocktail that could cause serious problems over the long run.

Don't assume that just because a product is sold in stores that it's safe to use. Here are some of the substances you may be putting in your mouth:

- **Dye.** Some artificial dyes used in toothpaste are a petroleum byproduct. These potentially carcinogenic synthetic compounds are readily absorbed by your lips and gums.
- **Fluoride.** Yes, sodium fluoride does help prevent tooth decay. It's also extremely toxic in large amounts. I don't know about you, but I don't really want to put something in my mouth that's used in pesticides and rat poison. Sodium fluoride is found in most commercial toothpastes.
- **Propylene Glycol.** Would you put antifreeze in your mouth and swish it around? Of course not, but some toothpastes contain this chemical, which has been classified as "Generally Recognized as Safe (GRAS)" by the FDA.
- **Sodium Lauryl Sulfate and Sodium Laureth Sulfate.** These detergents are added to

toothpaste to make it foam up. Most of the studies of these substances that have been done have consisted of using large dosages of the chemical over short periods of time. Studies have shown SLS to affect the recurrence of canker sores (54).

- **Triclosan.** The FDA states that triclosan is not known to be hazardous, but is currently reviewing its safety. Recent studies indicate it can cause cross-resistance to certain antibiotics (55) and may negatively impact the immune system and make allergies worse (56).

All these chemicals and more combine to make commercial mouthwash and toothpaste a potentially toxic choice over the long-term. Sure, you only get trace amounts of these chemicals each time you brush your teeth or rinse with mouthwash, but when you consider that most people use these products 3 to 5 times a day (or more), you've got the potential for serious long-term build-up.

You can make your own toothpaste at home using coconut oil, baking soda and essential oils that's every bit as effective as the stuff sold in stores.

Mix equal parts coconut oil and baking soda until a paste is formed. Stir in a few drops of an essential oil known to promote oral health like tea tree or eucalyptus oil and you've got toothpaste that's free of the many harmful chemicals mentioned above. Be aware that some people are sensitive to certain essential oils and can have allergic reactions, so proceed with caution. If your toothpaste isn't sweet enough, you can add a bit of Stevia to sweeten it up to your liking.

Oil pulling can also be used to soften up plaque and kill the bacteria that cause cavities. Oil pulling involves swishing coconut oil around the mouth like its mouthwash. Do this for 10 to 15 minutes and then rinse out your mouth with water. Whatever you do, don't swallow the coconut oil. It'll be full of nasty bacteria you don't want to eat.

Coconut oil also kills the candida bacteria that cause oral thrush. This painful infection causes white lesions to appear all over the tongue and mucus membranes in the mouth. Rinse your mouth with coconut oil twice a day to help kill the candida bacteria causing this infection.

Consult with an oral health specialist before starting use of coconut oil. There may be concerns you aren't aware of.

Adding Coconut Oil to Your Diet

First, a warning.

Coconut oil is packed full of fats that are gentle to most people's digestive systems and are easily digested by most people who try it. That said, a small percentage of the population can't handle consuming coconut oil because they are allergic to it or it doesn't agree with their digestive system. If you've never eaten coconut oil before and are attempting to add it to your diet, you should start off consuming a small amount first and go from there.

Take half a teaspoon the first time and wait for at least 4 hours to see if your digestive system and body react negatively to it. Then try a full teaspoon and wait for a reaction. After that, bump the dosage up to a tablespoon and then a couple tablespoons, each time waiting to see if there's a negative reaction.

If, at any time, you have a reaction, discontinue use immediately and consult with your physician.

There are a number of ways you can add coconut oil to your diet, and they're all easy. Here are some of the best ways to start eating coconut oil:

- **Replace vegetable oils and margarines with coconut oil.** You can usually make a 1:1 swap when switching coconut oil for other oils in your recipes. Coconut oil works especially well for baked goods because it adds a hint of sweetness to whatever it is you're baking.

- **Add a teaspoon or two to your smoothies.** Coconut oil blends well in smoothies and adds in a bit of coconut flavor.
- **Add it to hot drinks like coffee, tea or hot chocolate.** Coconut oil works well if you want to add a hint of sweetness to your warm drinks without adding extra sugar.
- **Use it to fry and sauté your foods.** If you insist on eating fried foods, coconut oil is less prone to oxidation and holds up well under high heat because of the saturated fat it contains.
- **Drizzle it on your salad.** A bit of coconut oil on your salad adds a hint of coconut to it and imparts an interesting flavor.
- **Replace butter on your popcorn.** Try adding coconut oil to your popcorn instead of butter. It tastes a lot better than it sounds.
- **Just eat it.** You can get an entire day's worth of coconut oil by taking three tablespoons of oil daily.
- **Use it to top ice cream.** Coconut oil tastes great drizzled over ice cream.

When it comes to adding coconut oil to your diet, use your imagination. Coconut oil is a versatile oil that can be used for a large number of applications in the kitchen.

Other Books You May Be Interested In

If you're interested in healthy eating, there are a number of other healthy foods you may be interested in adding to your diet. The following books may be of interest to you.

The Coconut Flour Cookbook: Delicious Gluten Free Coconut Flour Recipes

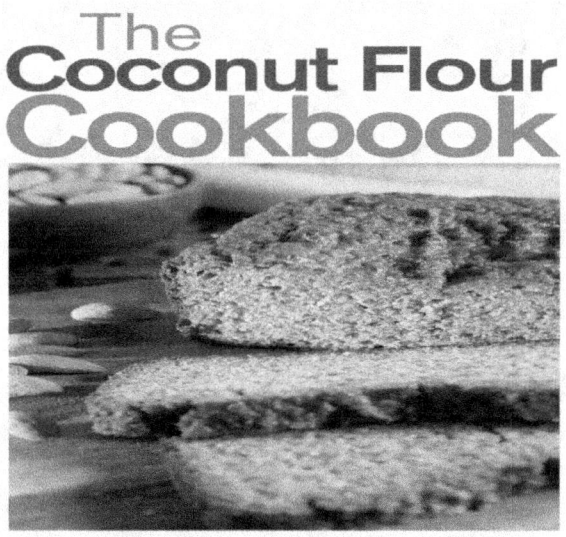

http://www.amazon.com/dp/B00CC0JFPM

The Almond Flour Cookbook: 30 Delicious and Gluten Free Recipes

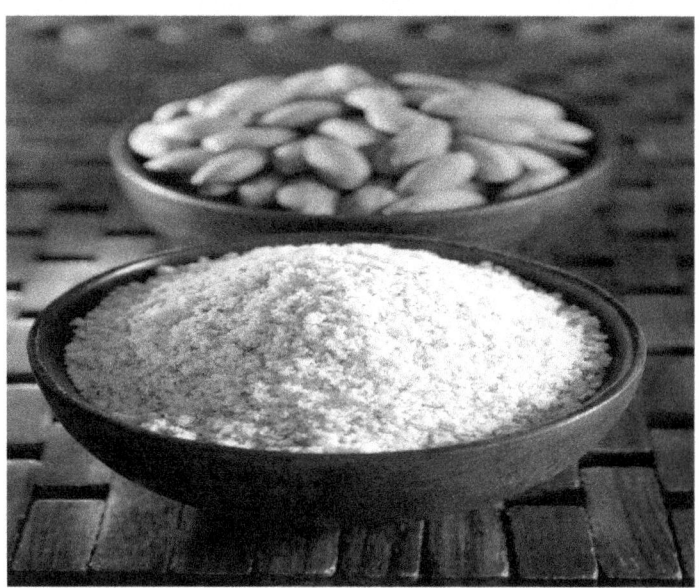

http://www.amazon.com/dp/B00CB3SJ0M

The Coconut Oil Guide: How to Stay Healthy, Lose Weight and Feel Good through Use of Coconut Oil

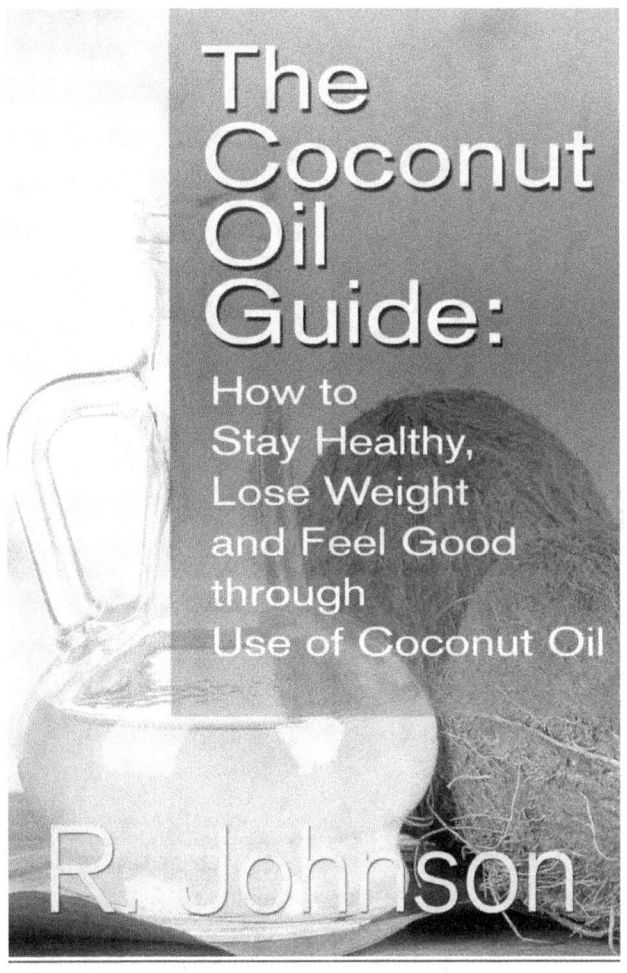

The Quinoa Cookbook: Healthy and Delicious Quinoa Recipes (Superfood Cookbooks)

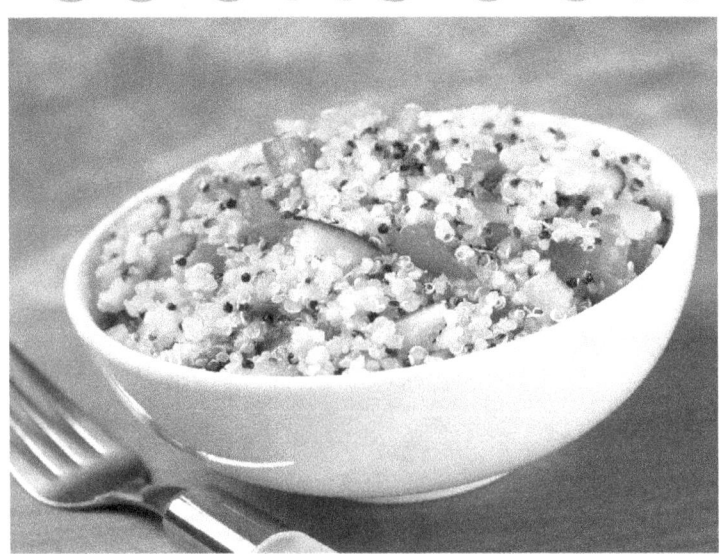

If you want information on essential oils and their applications, I recommend the following book:

The Aromatherapy & Essential Oils Handbook

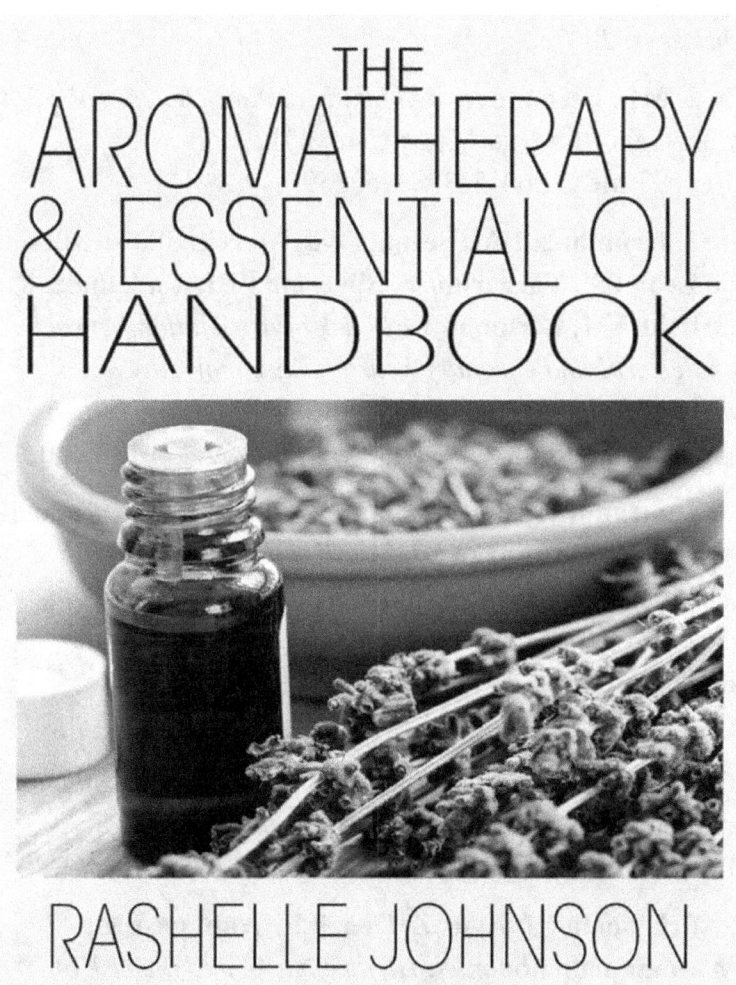

http://www.amazon.com/dp/B00BECCJXY

Works Cited

1. **Kavanagh K, Jones KL, Sawyer J, Kelley K, Carr JJ, Wagner JD, Rudel LL.** *Trans fat diet induces abdominal obesity and changes in insulin sensitivity in monkeys.* 2007.

2. **ML, Fernandez.** *Rethinking dietary cholesterol.* s.l. : Curr Opin Clin Nutr Metab Care, 2012. doi: 10.1097/MCO.0b013e32834d2259.

3. **Krumholz HM, Seeman TE, Merrill SS, Mendes de Leon CF, Vaccarino V, Silverman DI, Tsukahara R, Ostfeld AM, Berkman LF.** *Lack of association between cholesterol and coronary heart disease mortality and morbidity and all-cause mortality in persons older than 70 years.* New Haven, CT : JAMA, 1994. 272(17):1335-40..

4. **Strandberg TE, Salomaa VV, Naukkarinen VA, Vanhanen HT, Sarna SJ, Miettinen TA.** *Long-term mortality after 5-year multifactorial primary prevention of cardiovascular diseases in middle-aged men.* Helsinki, Finland : JAMA, 1991. 266(9):1225-9..

5. **Feranil AB, Duazo PL, Kuzawa CW, Adair LS.** *Coconut oil is associated with a beneficial lipid profile in pre-menopausal women in the Philippines.* Cebu City, Phillipines : Asia Pac J Clin Nutr, 2011. 20(2):190-5.

6. **Lipoeto NI, Agus Z, Oenzil F, Wahlqvist M, Wattanapenpaiboon N.** *Dietary intake and the risk of coronary heart disease among the coconut-consuming Minangkabau in West Sumatra, Indonesia.* Padang, West Sumatra : Asia Pac J Clin Nutr, 2004. 13(4):377-84.

7. **Assunção ML, Ferreira HS, dos Santos AF, Cabral CR Jr, Florêncio TM.** *Effects of dietary coconut oil on the biochemical and anthropometric profiles of women presenting abdominal obesity.* Maceió, Brazil : Lipids, 2009 May 13. doi: 10.1007/s11745-009-3306-6.

8. *Dietary polyunsaturated fatty acids and composition of human aortic plaques.* **Felton CV, Crook D, Davies MJ, Oliver MF.** Oct., 1994, Lancet, pp. 29;344(8931):1195-6.

9. **Zeman M, Jirak R, Vecka M, Raboch J, Zak A.** *N-3 polyunsaturated fatty acids in psychiatric diseases: mechanisms and clinical data.* s.l. : Neuro Endocrinol Lett., 2012.

10. **Dahm CC, Gorst-Rasmussen A, Crowe FL, Roswall N, Tjønneland A, Drogan D, Boeing H, Teucher B, Kaaks R, Adarakis G, Zylis D, Trichopoulou A, Fedirko V, Chajes V, Jenab M, Palli D, Pala V, Tumino R, Ricceri F, van Kranen H, Bueno-de-Mesquita HB, Quirós JR,.** *Fatty acid patterns and risk of prostate cancer in a case-control study nested within the European Prospective Investigation into Cancer and Nutrition.* Department of Cardiology, Center for Cardiovascular Research. Aalborg, Denmark : s.n., 2012.

11. **Simopoulos AP.** *The importance of the ratio of omega-6/omega-3 essential fatty acids.* Washington, D.C. : Biomed Pharmacother, Oct. 2002.

12. *Dietary fat intake and risk of type 2 diabetes in women.* **Salmerón J, Hu FB, Manson JE, et al.** 2001, Am J Clin Nutr , pp. 73:1019–26.

13. *The solid fat content of stearic acid-rich fats determines their postprandial effects.* **Berry SEE, Miller GJ, Sanders TAB.** s.l. : Am J Clin Nutr , 2007, Am J Clin Nutr , p. 85.

14. *Atherosclerosis: a problem in newer public health.* **A, KEYS.** 1953.

15. **National Heart, Lung, and Blood Institute (NHLBI).** News from the Women's Health Initiative: Reducing Total Fat Intake May Have Small Effect on Risk of Breast Cancer, No Effect on Risk of Colorectal Cancer, Heart Disease, or Stroke . *NIH News.* [Online] February 7, 2006. [Cited: April 21, 2013.] http://www.nih.gov/news/pr/feb2006/nhlbi-07.htm.

16. *Concerning the possibility of a nut...* **Castelli, William P.** July 1992, Archives of Internal Medicine.

17. *Dietary intakes of polyunsaturated fatty acids and indices of oxidative stress in human volunteers.* **A Jenkinson, M F Franklin, K Wahle and G G Duthie.** 7, July 1999, European Journal of Clinical Nutrition, Vol. 53, pp. 523-528.

18. *Results analysis of clinical HIV trial with monoglycerides [presentation].* **Tayag E, Dayrit CS.** Chennai, India : The 37th Cocotech Meeting, July 25, 2000.

19. **Zakaria ZA, Somchit MN, Mat Jais AM, Teh LK, Salleh MZ, Long K.** *In vivo Antinociceptive and Anti-inflammatory Activities of Dried and Fermented Processed Virgin Coconut Oil.* s.l. : Med Princ Pract., 2011 March. 20(3):231-6. Epub.

20. **Kono H, Fujii H, Asakawa M, Maki A, Amemiya H, Hirai Y, Matsuda M, Yamamoto M.** *Medium-chain triglycerides enhance secretory IgA expression in rat intestine after administration of endotoxin.* s.l. : Am J Physiol Gastrointest Liver Physiol, 2004 June. 286(6):G1081-9.

21. **S Intahphuak, P Khonsung, A Panthong.** *Coconut oil has anti-inflammatory, analgesic and antipyretic activities.* s.l. : Pharm Biol, 2010 February. 48(2):151-7. PMID: 20645831.

22. *Meal triacylglycerol profile modulates postprandial absorption of carotenoids in humans.* **Shellen R. Goltz, Wayne W. Campbell, Chureeporn Chitchumroonchokchai, Mark L. Falla, Mario G. Ferruzi.** 6, s.l. : Molecular Nutrition & Food Research, 2012 June, Vol. 56, pp. 866-877. DOI: 10.1002/mnfr.201100687.

23. *Coconut Oil Enhances Tomato Carotenoid Tissue Accumulation Compared to Safflower Oil in the Mongolian Gerbil (Meriones unguiculatus).* **Conlon LE, King RD, Moran NE, Erdman JW Jr.** s.l. : J Agric Food Chem, 2012 August. [Epub ahead of print] PubMed PMID: 22866697.

24. **Tianyao Huo, Steven J. Schwartz and Mark L. Failla.** *Impact of Fatty Acid Chain Length and Saturation on Micellarization of Carotenoids during.* s.l. : Ohio State University Interdisciplinary Ph.D. Program in Nutrition. http://hdl.handle.net/1811/6149 .

25. **Cabré E, Gassull MA.** *Nutritional and metabolic issues in inflammatory bowel disease.* Catalonia, Spain : Curr Opin Clin Nutr Metab Care, 2003 September. 6(5):569-76.

26. **Canaris GJ, Manowitz NR, Mayor G, Ridgway EC.** *The Colorado thyroid disease prevalence study.* s.l. : Arch Intern Med, 2000. 160:526-34.

27. **Gupta V, Walia L, Gupta S, Bajwa N.** Comparison of the Effects of Coconut Oil and Soyabean Oil on TSH Level and Weight Gain in Rabbits. *Online J Health Allied Scs.* [Online] 2009. [Cited: April 5, 2013.] http://www.ojhas.org/issue29/2009-1-7.htm.

28. **Hill JO, Peters JC, Yang D, Sharp T, Kaler M, Abumrad NN, Greene HL.** *Thermogenesis in humans during overfeeding with medium-chain triglycerides.* Nashville, TN : Metabolism, 1989 Jul. 38(7):641-8.

29. **St-Onge MP, Ross R, Parsons WD, Jones PJ.** *Medium-chain triglycerides increase energy expenditure and decrease adiposity in overweight men.* Ste-Anne-de-Bellevue, Quebec, Canada : Obes Res, 2003 March. 395-402.

30. **Seaton TB, Welle SL, Warenko MK, Campbell RG.** *Thermic effect of medium-chain and long-chain triglycerides in man.* s.l. : Am J Clin Nutr, 1986 November. 44(5):630-4.

31. **Adam M Persky, N Seth Berry, Gary M Pollack, and Kim L R Brouwer.** *Modelling the cardiovascular effects of ephedrine.* s.l. : Br J Clin Pharmacol, 2004 May. 57(5): 552–562.

32. **ABERER, W, et al., et al.** *PROPYLENE-GLYCOL - CUTANEOUS SIDE-EFFECTS AND TEST METHODS - LITERATURE AND RESULTS OF A MULTICENTER STUDY OF THE GERMAN CONTACT ALLERGY GROUP.* s.l. : DERMATOSEN BERUF UMWELT, 1993. 41(1): 25-27.

33. **Verallo-Rowell VM, Dillague KM, Syah-Tjundawan BS.** *Novel antibacterial and emollient effects of coconut and virgin olive oils in adult atopic dermatitis.* s.l. : Dermatitis, 2008 November - December. 19(6):308-15..

34. **Nakatsuji T, Kao MC, Fang JY, Zouboulis CC, Zhang L, Gallo RL, Huang CM.** *Antimicrobial property of lauric acid against Propionibacterium acnes: its therapeutic potential for inflammatory acne vulgaris.* San Diego, CA : J Invest Dermatol, 2009 October. 129(10):2480-8. doi: 10.1038/jid.2009.93. Epub 2009 Apr 23.

35. **Agero AL, Verallo-Rowell VM.** *A randomized double-blind controlled trial comparing extra virgin coconut oil with mineral oil as a moisturizer for mild to moderate xerosis.* Makati City, Phillipines : Dermatitis, 2004 September. 15(3):109-16.

36. **Nevin KG, Rajamohan T.** *Effect of topical application of virgin coconut oil on skin components and antioxidant status during dermal wound healing in young rats.* s.l. : Skin Pharmacol Physiol, 2010. 23(6):290-7. doi: 10.1159/000313516. Epub 2010 Jun 3.

37. **D.O. Ogbolu, A.A. Oni, O.A. Daini and A.P. Oloko1.** *In Vitro Antimicrobial Properties of Coconut Oil on Candida Species in.* s.l. : Mary Ann Liebert, Inc. and Korean Society of Food Science and Nutrition, 2007. DOI: 10.1089/jmf.2006.1209.

38. **Yang D, Pornpattananangkul D, Nakatsuji T, Chan M, Carson D, Huang CM, Zhang L.** *The antimicrobial activity of liposomal lauric acids against Propionibacterium acnes.* s.l. : Biomaterials, 2009 October. doi: 10.1016/j.biomaterials.2009.07.033. Epub 2009 Aug 8.

39. **Logan, Whitney P Bowe and Alan C.** *Acne vulgaris, probiotics and the gut-brain-skin axis - back to the future?* s.l. : Gut Pathogens, 2011 January. doi:10.1186/1757-4749-3-1.

40. **Rele AS, Mohile RB.** *Effect of mineral oil, sunflower oil, and coconut oil on prevention of hair damage.* Mumbai, India : Journal of Cosmetic Science, 2003 March - April. 54(2):175-92.

41. **Ruetsch SB, Kamath YK, Rele AS, Mohile RB.** *Secondary ion mass spectrometric investigation of penetration of coconut and mineral oils into human hair fibers: relevance to hair damage.* Princeton, NJ : Journal of Cosmetic Science, 2001 May - June. 52(3):169-84.

42. **AARTI S. RELE and R. B. MOHILE.** *Effect of coconut oil on prevention of hair damage. Part I.* s.l. : Journal of Cosmetic Science, 1999 September. 50, 327-339.

43. **Burgess IF, Brunton ER, Burgess NA.** *Clinical trial showing superiority of a coconut and anise spray over*

permethrin 0.43% lotion for head louse infestation.
Cambridge, UK : Eur J Pediatr., 2010 Jan. 169(1):55-62.
doi: 10.1007/s00431-009-0978-0. Epub 2009 Apr 3.

44. **Lim EL, Hollingsworth KG, Aribisala BS, Chen
MJ, Mathers JC, Taylor R.** *Reversal of type 2 diabetes:
normalisation of beta cell function in association with
decreased pancreas and liver triacylglycerol.* Newcastle :
Diabetologia, 2011 October. doi: 10.1007/s00125-011-
2204-7. Epub 2011 Jun 9.

45. **Kochikuzhyil BM, Devi K, Fattepur SR.** *Effect of
saturated fatty acid-rich dietary vegetable oils on lipid
profile, antioxidant enzymes and glucose tolerance in
diabetic rats.* Bangalor, India : Indian J Pharmacol, 2010
June. 42(3):142-5. doi: 10.4103/0253-7613.66835.

46. **Eckel RH, Hanson AS, Chen AY, Berman JN,
Yost TJ, Brass EP.** *Dietary substitution of medium-chain
triglycerides improves insulin-mediated glucose
metabolism in NIDDM subjects.* Denver : Diabetes, 1992
May. 41(5):641-7.

47. **Bassett CN, Montine TJ.** *Lipoproteins and lipid
peroxidation in Alzheimer's disease.* Alabama : J Nutr
Health Aging, 2003. 7(1):24-9.

48. **Seneff S, Wainwright G, Mascitelli L.** *Nutrition
and Alzheimer's disease: the detrimental role of a high
carbohydrate diet.* MA : Eur J Intern Med, 2011 April. doi:
10.1016/j.ejim.2010.12.017. Epub 2011 Jan 26.

49. **Kalpana P. Padala, MD, MS, et al., et al.** *The
Effect of HMG-CoA Reductase Inhibitors on Cognition in
Patients With Alzheimer's Dementia.* Little Rock, AR : The

American Journal of Geriatric Pharmacotherapy, 2012 Oct. doi: 10.1016/j.amjopharm.2012.08.002. Epub 2012 Aug 22..

50. *A comparison of long-chain triglycerides and medium-chain triglycerides on weight loss and tumour size in a cachexia model.* **M. J. Tisdale, R. A. Brennan.** s.l. : Br J Cancer, 1988, Vols. November; 58(5): 580–583. .

51. **Cohen LA, Thompson DO, Maeura Y, Weisburger JH.** *Influence of dietary medium-chain triglycerides on the development of N-methylnitrosourea-induced rat mammary tumors.* s.l. : Cancer Res., 1984 Nov. 44(11):5023-8.

52. **Carroll KK, Khor HT.** *Effects of level and type of dietary fat on of mammary tumors induced in female Sprague-Dawley rats by 7, 12-dimethylbenz(a)anthracene.* s.l. : Lipids, 1971. 6:415-20.

53. *Dietary polyunsaturated fat in relation to mammary carcinogenesis in rats.* **Laura M. Braden.** 4, s.l. : Lipids, April 1986, Vol. 21. 285-288.

54. **P, Herlofson BB. Barkvoll.** *Sodium lauryl sulfate and recurrent aphthous ulcers.* s.l. : Acta Odontol Scand, 1994. 52: 257-259. Oslo. ISSN 0001-6357.

55. **Schweizer, Herbert P.** *Triclosan: a widely used biocide and its link to antibiotics.* s.l. : FEMS Microbiology Letters, 2006 January. DOI: 10.1111/j.1574-6968.2001.tb10772.x.

56. **Erin M. Rees Clayton, Megan Todd, Jennifer Beam Dowd, Allison E. Aiello.** *The Impact of Bisphenol A*

and Triclosan on Immune Parameters in the U.S. Population, NHANES 2003–2006. s.l. : Environ Health Perspect, 2010. pp. 119:390-396.

57. **OIL WORLD Publications.** *Oil World Annual 2006.* Hamburg, Germany : ISTA Mielke GmbH, 2006. Langenberg 25, 21077.